Biohacking Breakthroughs

The Ultimate Guide to Unleashing Your Potential for Optimal Health, Performance, and Success

Olivia Rivers

© **Copyright 2023 - All rights reserved.**

The content contained within this book may not be reproduced, duplicated, or transmitted without direct written permission from the author or the publisher.

Under no circumstances will any blame or legal responsibility be held against the publisher, or author, for any damages, reparation, or monetary loss due to the information contained within this book, either directly or indirectly.

Legal Notice:

This book is copyright protected. It is only for personal use. You cannot amend, distribute, sell, use, quote or paraphrase any part, or the content within this book, without the consent of the author or publisher.

Disclaimer Notice:

Please note the information contained within this document is for educational and entertainment purposes only. All effort has been executed to present accurate, up to date, reliable, complete information. No warranties of any kind are declared or implied. Readers acknowledge that the author is not engaged in the rendering of legal, financial, medical, or professional advice. The content within this book has been derived from various sources. Please consult a licensed professional before attempting any techniques outlined in this book.

By reading this document, the reader agrees that under no circumstances is the author responsible for any losses, direct or indirect, that are incurred as a result of the use of the information contained within this document, including, but not limited to, errors, omissions, or inaccuracies.

Empower Your Journey with the Biohacking Planner

Unleash the full potential of your biohacking journey with our exclusive Biohacking planner.

By downloading and printing this essential tool, you'll embark on a transformative path to peak performance and unparalleled well-being.

This planner is your guide to optimizing every aspect of your life, empowering you to maximize energy, focus, and vitality.

Scan the QR code and follow the instructions to ignite your journey towards holistic optimization and relentless fulfilment.

Your Empowering biohacking transformation starts here.

Table of Contents

INTRODUCTION 1

CHAPTER 1: UNDERSTANDING BIOHACKING 5

WHAT IS BIOHACKING AND ITS CORE PRINCIPLES? 5
   Core Principles of Biohacking 5
   Exploring Technology-Based Biohacking 7
UNLEASHING YOUR TRUE POTENTIAL WITH BIOHACKING 8
   From Ordinary to Extraordinary 8
   Discovering Hidden Capabilities 10
THE MINDSET SHIFT 10
   Power in Your Hands 11
   Being Receptive to Change 11
DEBUNKING COMMON MISCONCEPTIONS ABOUT BIOHACKING 12
   Biohacking Is Dangerous and Illegal 12
   All Biohacking Methods Are Reliable and Safe 12
   Only Scientists and Tech Wizards Can Biohack 13
   Biohacking Is All about Supplements and Nootropics 14
   Biohacking Provides Immediate Results 14
   Biohacks Are the Same for Everyone 15
   All Biohacking Methods Are Supported by Science 15
REAL-LIFE SUCCESS STORIES 15

CHAPTER 2: BIOHACKING FOR OPTIMAL NUTRITION 17

THE ROLE OF NUTRITION IN BIOHACKING 17
   The Importance of Gut Health 18
REVOLUTIONIZE YOUR DIET 19
   Developing Healthy Eating Habits 19
   How to Change Your Diet 21
BIOHACKING YOUR PLATE 23
   Knowing Your Macro and Micronutrients 23
   What Should Your Plate Look Like? 26
DESIGNING A BIOHACKING DIET FOR IMPROVED ENERGY, FOCUS, AND VITALITY .. 27

Elimination Diet 27
Intermittent Fasting 30
Ketogenic Diet 31
Paleo Diet 33
Cut Out Processed Sugars 33
Let Go of Toxic Consumption 35
STRATEGIES FOR PERSONALIZING YOUR NUTRITION PLAN AND OPTIMIZING NUTRIENT ABSORPTION.. 37
Try Different Diets... 37
Make Use of a Food Journal 38

CHAPTER 3: MASTERING SLEEP AND RECOVERY 41

THE IMPORTANCE OF SUFFICIENT SLEEP... 41
WHY RECOVERY IS CRUCIAL FOR BIOHACKING 43
BIOHACKING SLEEP 45
Biohacking Insomnia... 45
Hacking Your Circadian Rhythm 47
Biohacking Devices and Resources to Use 49
PRACTICAL TIPS FOR ENHANCING RECOVERY AND PHYSICAL PERFORMANCE......... 50
Prioritizing Muscle Recovery... 50
Nourish Your Body 52
Have Rest Days 52

CHAPTER 4: BOOSTING COGNITIVE ABILITIES AND MENTAL PERFORMANCE 55

BIOHACKING THE BRAIN FOR IMPROVED COGNITIVE FUNCTION 56
Understanding the Brain Structure and How it Functions 56
Diet to Fulfill Your Nutritional Needs... 57
Supplements to Try 58
Using Nootropics for Cognitive Advancement 60
NOOTROPICS, SUPPLEMENTS, AND TECHNIQUES FOR ENHANCING FOCUS, MEMORY, AND CREATIVITY 61
The Various Uses for Supplements 62
The Value of Nootropics 63
How to Use Nootropics and Supplements Effectively 64
Types of Nootropics 68
MINDFULNESS PRACTICES AND MEDITATION FOR MENTAL CLARITY AND CALMNESS 70
Practicing Mindfulness 71
Practicing Meditation 72
ENHANCING COGNITIVE BEHAVIOR WITH TECHNOLOGY 74

Neurofeedback 74
Brain Simulation 75
Cognitive Training Apps 75

CHAPTER 5: MANAGING STRESS AND OPTIMIZING EMOTIONAL AND MENTAL WELL-BEING 77

THE RELATIONSHIP BETWEEN STRESS AND BIOHACKING 78
The Impact of Stress on the Mind 78
The Impact of Stress on The Body 79
EFFECTIVE STRESS MANAGEMENT TECHNIQUES 80
Embrace Nature 81
Meditation 82
Aromatherapy 84
Breathwork 87
Use a Journal 89

CHAPTER 6: BIOHACKING FOR LONGEVITY AND HEALTHY AGING 91

EXPLORING THE RELATIONSHIP BETWEEN BIOHACKING AND LONGEVITY 91
Living a Life of Longevity 92
Aging Gracefully 92
ANTI-AGING APPROACHES, CELLULAR OPTIMIZATION, AND METHODS FOR PROMOTING HEALTHY AGING 94
Lifestyle Factors That Contribute to a Long Life 94
Hormone Replacement Therapy 97
Exploring Cutting Edge Technology 98

CHAPTER 7: PERSONALIZING YOUR BIOHACKING ROUTINE 101

CUSTOMIZING YOUR BIOHACKING ROUTINE 101
Identify Your Personal Goals 102
Experiment with Biohacking and Your Body 104
Trial and Error 105
Download Your Planner 106

CHAPTER 8: ADVANCED BIOHACKING TECHNOLOGIES AND TRENDS 107

EXPLORING CUTTING-EDGE BIOHACKING TECHNOLOGIES, GADGETS, PRACTICES, AND DEVICES. 107
Biohacking Blood Tests 108
Wearable Technology 110
Cold and Heat Therapy 110
High Intensity Interval Training (HIIT) 111
Biofeedback 111

Integrating Science Fiction with Reality 112
   Using Artificial Intelligence and Virtual Reality 113
   Cyborg Biohacking 114
   Nanotechnology 114
   Exploring Human Microchipping 115
Evaluating the Potential Benefits and Risks of Advanced Biohacking Techniques 116
   Understanding the Potential Benefits 117
   Uncovering the Risk Factors 118
   Real-World Applications of Biohacking Technologies 119

CHAPTER 9: IMPLEMENTING BIOHACKING IN YOUR DAILY LIFE 123

Practical Tips for Integrating Biohacking into Your Daily Routine..... 123
   Build Your Biohacking Lifestyle 124
Overcoming Common Challenges and Obstacles................................ 126
   Give it Time 126
   Trying New Biohacks 127
   Adjusting to Change 127
   Resisting Tempting Bad Habits 129
   Strengthening Your Mind and Body Connection 131

CONCLUSION 133

REFERENCES 139

Introduction

What if you were told you could completely transform the way you feel, your quality of life, daily performance, and physical and mental capacity, by simply hacking your body with specific techniques? You may think that this sounds too good to be true, but I'm here to tell you that it is more than achievable with biohacking.

Life can be extremely overwhelming and demanding, which can result in us neglecting our holistic well-being. It can be so easy to get stuck in an unhealthy routine, especially when you aren't mindful of what you consume and the habits you practice. Once you find a healthy routine through biohacking, you'll be able to live a higher quality of life that leaves you feeling satisfied, happy, and healthy.

If you're looking to enhance your physical abilities, drastically improve your physical well-being, or even balance your emotional and mental wellness, you're in the right place! This book explores all the ways you can strive for self-improvement by modifying your eating habits, optimizing your sleep, and exposing yourself to modern techniques and supplements.

But what makes biohacking so effective? It's a modern and scientific approach to achieving self-improvement, as you explore innovations, cutting-edge technologies, and scientific advances. By prioritizing nutrition and gut health, you're able to develop healthy and studied habits that are proven to boost your cognitive abilities, physical performance, and everyday functioning. You'll also find that your emotional and mental well-being is enhanced, as your mind and body work harmoniously as one.

We will discuss some of the most recent scientific breakthroughs in biohacking and expose both the pros and cons of certain techniques. Before embarking on this journey, it's crucial for you to be aware of ethical practices and some of the dangers and misconceptions you can face with biohacking. Knowing where to find your reliable biohacking news and updates can ensure that you have the right resources to continue this transformation journey after completing this book.

Biohacking focuses on patterns, experimentation, and repetition. You learn how to hack your mind and body, by adapting to specific strategies and techniques that are suitable for the functioning of your holistic being. Before you pursue this journey, it's crucial for you to have an open and receptive mind to change. You're going to be exposed to a lot of change within your habits, thoughts, and eating patterns, which can be challenging to adjust to at first. When you practice these healthy and enriching habits every day, you will find that over time it becomes second nature for you. So, as you explore this journey, be patient with yourself and realistic with your results.

Throughout this book we will explore ways for you to address health conditions, weight management issues, and alternative ways to nourish and look after your body. You'll be provided with practical and efficient step-by-step guides that allow you to practice biohacking in the most accurate way possible.

We all want to live long and healthy lives, and this is possible when you start your biohacking journey now. Regardless of what age you are, the stage of life you're currently in, or the goals that you have for your mind and body, you can benefit greatly from biohacking. If you're older, biohacking can help you to slow down the aging process. As an athlete, biohacking can allow you to unlock all of your health and fitness capabilities. Health enthusiasts can discover new techniques and strategies to further enhance physical health. If you're a career-driven professional or entrepreneur, you will be guided to maximize your productivity, mental clarity, and cognitive behavior. As a science enthusiast, you can indulge in the integration of human and science. If you simply want to be a high achiever in your life, exploring *Biohacking Breakthroughs* will encourage motivation, health, and a happy, successful life.

Whether you're a beginner who is being introduced to biohacking and its techniques, or you're someone who already practices biohacking, and you want to expand your knowledge and skills, *Biohacking Breakthroughs* will provide you with the guidance you need to optimize your life through groundbreaking technology.

It's time to embrace technology, as it's the way forward for our future. Using wearable devices, trying out efficient apps, and integrating technology into your everyday life will enhance your biohacking experience. It's fascinating to be aware of all the remarkable things technology can achieve through us in our lives. Be open to the unique practices and strategies you'll practice for your body along this journey, as personalized routines will lead you to optimal success. All of our minds and bodies are different, so we should treat them with special care!

Chapter 1:

Understanding Biohacking

The world of biohacking is remarkable. It provides you with the opportunity to become the best, healthiest version of yourself through practical strategies and techniques. You have the power to advance your physical fitness, wellness, and abilities, all through successful and mindful biohacking. The potential is within you to transform your biological capabilities; it's time to learn more about biohacking so you can turn it into your reality!

What Is Biohacking and Its Core Principles?

Biohacking is a practice that works on enhancing your mind and body through biological hacks and strategies that are most suitable for you. It uses fresh and modern innovations to unlock your body's full biological potential. If you are seeking self-improvement or you feel as though you're missing something to become the best version of yourself, biohacking will provide you with the positive change that you need.

Core Principles of Biohacking

The world of biohacking can be viewed as controversial to many, as it's a methodology that allows you to cheat the system of life. You spin back the clock on your body and enhance it in unfathomable ways. The core principles of biohacking showcase the true nature of this practice, which can be seen as positive and enriching:

- **Putting your health and safety first.** Biohacking is all about considering your health and safety. It's crucial to practice biohacking strategies that prioritize this principle, as its main objective should be to better your overall health.

- **Living long healthy lives.** The objective of biohacking is to increase your lifespan as much as you can. You want to be able to live a fulfilling lifestyle in your twenties and your eighties. We can often assume that once you reach old age, your life is over, and you can no longer pursue a lifestyle that makes you happy. In reality, this couldn't be further from the truth, as being healthy allows you to live a long and fulfilling life, even when you're approaching your nineties.

- **Unlocking full potential.** Many people go through life not realizing all of the untapped potential they have within them. They settle for the way they are, which causes them to neglect all of the hidden skills and talents that they could master with biological enrichment. Biohacking explores all of your greatest strengths and abilities, whether they are hidden or evident. This allows you to advance your best qualities and unlock your potential mentally, physically, and emotionally.

These core principles focus on the well-being of an individual, as it's all about living a healthy and successful life that makes you feel content. As you embrace biohacking and its various practices, keep these core principles in mind, as it will prioritize your own benefit. This is a methodology that isn't just about reaching physical goals, as you experience internal and external growth along the way.

Exploring Technology-Based Biohacking

Of course, when we talk about biohacking, we also need to explore some of the technology-based techniques and strategies that this methodology uses. The essence of biohacking is embracing modern trends and studies to enrich your wellness routines. Technology plays a big role in our present and future lives, so it's only fitting to include it in your new biohacking routine:

- **Apps.** New apps are being published every day. There are a variety of apps with different functions that can provide you with your specific needs along your journey. If you need to stay more organized, you can find an app that helps you to stay organized. If accountability is something you struggle with when embracing change, you can download an app that reminds you to stay on track and keeps you accountable for your actions.

- **Wearable devices.** Wearing devices like Fitbits, Apple Watches, and AirTags can help you to reach your fitness goals and potential. These are devices that help you to track your movement, goals, and daily achievements. Having these will keep you motivated to continuously work to achieve the goals you've set for yourself. For example, an Apple Watch, or its equivalent, can help you track the number of steps you walk in a day. If your biohacking goal is to walk 10,000 steps a day, your wearable device can remind you of how many steps you need to do, and you'll receive a notification when you accomplish this goal.

- **Embedded implants.** Technology is becoming more and more advanced, so much so that we are entering an era of embedded implants. Though this is a very controversial topic, biohacking explores all possibilities of technological advancements and innovations. Some embedded implant technology that's in the market includes magnetic implants, memory chips, and GPS systems.

When you use technology to your advantage, you will discover how much you're able to accomplish. Take advantage of these opportunities at your disposal so that you can find out new techniques and strategies that work for you. Many people may view the rise of technology as something negative, as our devices can be really distracting and time-consuming.

Unleashing Your True Potential with Biohacking

Our bodies have so much potential to reach optimal health, fitness, and happiness. It's time for you to unleash all of this untapped potential through the power of biohacking. You can reach new heights in your physical abilities, achieve greater motivation and accomplishments in your career, and wake up feeling like the best version of yourself every morning.

From Ordinary to Extraordinary

Being able to escape the ordinary through biohacking will allow you to achieve the extraordinary. Living with mediocrity and basic levels of health and happiness can be sufficient, but what if you could explore a more thrilling and satisfying life for yourself? Practicing this methodology can help you to escape your ordinary lifestyle in the following ways:

- **Peak physical performance.** If you're an athlete, being able to achieve your peak physical performance can allow you to achieve great things in your career. When you have personal physical goals, biohacking can help you to achieve them. Even if you aren't an athlete and you don't care much for physical activity, prioritizing biohacking can allow you to unleash physical abilities you never knew you had.

- **Mental sharpness.** If focusing and completing tasks is something you struggle with, developing mental sharpness will drastically boost your abilities. This can allow you to excel in various aspects of your life, as your sharpness helps you to make better decisions, accomplish tasks and responsibilities in time, and impress colleagues and bosses in your professional life.

- **Emotional relief and stability.** When you're living an ordinary life without being mindful of the foods you consume, the habits you practice, and the way you treat your body, you may find yourself experiencing a lot of emotional fluctuation. Life can be really overwhelming, which can fill you with a variety of negative emotions like stress, sadness, and frustration. Hacking your way to becoming the best version of yourself will allow you to feel a lot more stable and happier emotionally.

Being the best version of yourself while living a day-to-day life that is rewarding can be a fulfilling experience. You gain confidence and self-esteem when you find yourself excelling in various aspects of your life. Living an extraordinary life can expose you to so many unique and thrilling experiences that you would have never tried before starting this journey.

Discovering Hidden Capabilities

As you embark on this transformation, you will be surprised to discover how many hidden capabilities and strengths you have. There is so much untapped potential within you that you haven't been able to explore because of your unhealthy habits and routines. Once you completely change how you fuel and look after your mind and body, you will discover all of these new characteristics and abilities you have.

Discovering that you can do more than you thought you could can be a really exciting realization. You're so impressed by these new skills that you find ways to apply them to your everyday life. You'll be able to integrate these new skills and abilities through various aspects of your life. For example, if you discover that you're able to run for a long distance without stopping, you may consider running a marathon. This can be a huge achievement that brings you lots of enjoyment and health benefits.

The Mindset Shift

In order to experience optimal success from your biohacking journey, you need to be able to transform your mindset. When you put your mind to it along this journey, you will be able to achieve groundbreaking results. Believing in yourself and your capabilities to get certain tasks done and goals accomplished, will give you the motivation and willpower you need to achieve a lifestyle that makes you happy!

Your mindset contributes to your daily thoughts, behavior, and decisions. Our minds can often work on autopilot as we experience our day-to-day lives. When you work on shifting your mindset, you can find it easier to adapt to a lifestyle and daily routine that ensures your overall well-being and happiness. Your mindset can either block you or motivate you along this journey, so knowing how to adapt it for your necessary circumstances will allow you to achieve success in your life.

Power in Your Hands

As much as life can be overwhelming and unpredictable, you are in control of your own health and well-being. If you're constantly waiting to be less busy, for the circumstances in your life to be better, or for a golden opportunity, you will wait forever to start this journey. The power is in your hands, so it's time to pursue biohacking now, regardless of what's going on in your life.

You also need to remember that you have power to transform yourself or your lifestyle in a way that makes you happy and healthy. Be confident in yourself to achieve the changes that you require to fulfill healthy growth and development. You are capable of adapting to a new lifestyle that nourishes both your mind and body.

Being Receptive to Change

When you're working on shifting your mindset, you need to consider how open-minded you are. One of the most challenging aspects of this journey is that you have to experience a lot of change. It can be challenging to welcome change into your life, especially when you've grown so familiar with how you traditionally fulfill certain habits and everyday tasks.

Unfortunately, staying within your comfort zone and practicing the habits that are familiar to you won't help you to grow. You need to be brave and daring, by pushing yourself outside of your comfort zone and welcoming change into your life. It's this change that will allow you to live a more satisfying and enjoyable lifestyle.

Debunking Common Misconceptions about Biohacking

As with most things in life, there are usually misconceptions and myths that can deter you from exploring this journey. It's important for you to have a realistic and accurate representation of biohacking and all it has to offer. Don't let these myths and misconceptions prevent you from pursuing a practice that will allow your mind and body to thrive.

Biohacking Is Dangerous and Illegal

Many critics have a misconception that biohacking is a dangerous and harmful practice that should be illegal. This couldn't be further from the truth. Though there are some factors of biohacking that are illegal like DIY engineering, most regular biohacking practices are safe and legal to use.

All Biohacking Methods Are Reliable and Safe

As much as biohacking as a whole is safe and legal, there are some harmful methods you should look out for in this field. Some biohacking tips out there may seem legitimate, but if you practice them, they could actually decrease your health and overall quality of life. As we discussed in the previous misconception, there are certain biohacking practices that give this methodology a bad name.

Unfortunately, some biohackers want to use their illegitimate methods and practices to attract people for their own benefit. This is why it's so crucial for you to be aware of where you resource your biohacking information from. Ensure that it is an accredited individual, and if their techniques and strategies seem a bit suspicious, do your own research before practicing them. Trust your gut and do your own research and you won't find yourself following harmful biohacks.

Only Scientists and Tech Wizards Can Biohack

Many people believe that because biohacking is a scientific practice, it can only be successfully used by scientists and tech wizards. You think that it's too technical for you to understand or practice. What's important to remember is that biohacking is for absolutely everyone. Whether you have experience in this world or you are learning about all of these innovations for the first time, biohacking is easily accessible to you.

There are some specialized techniques and strategies, which we will discuss later, that should be practiced when you have more experience and knowledge as a biohacker. With this being said, most biohacking practices are straightforward and accessible to everyone, but it does take commitment and hard work to make it a way of life for you. You don't need to be a scientist or tech wizard to be a biohacker, but you do need to have the strength and willpower to change your lifestyle routine for the better.

Biohacking Is All about Supplements and Nootropics

Though supplements, nootropics, and 'smart drugs' make up a part of biohacking, it isn't the main focus of this practice. The focal point of biohacking isn't centered around the supplements and nootropics you consume, as it is a very versatile practice. We will explore the various supplements you can consider along this journey, as it will enhance your experience, but it's important to remember that biohacking is about a lot more than just supplements.

It's a holistic lifestyle change, which will require lots of action and participation. Biohacking is more about applying suitable hacks and practices to your day-to-day life that will unlock your biological capabilities.

Biohacking Provides Immediate Results

If you're looking for a quick fix with your mind and body, biohacking isn't your solution. Biohacking can provide you with the most groundbreaking, long-term, and rewarding results, but it does take time to achieve them. To truly benefit from biohacking, you need to use the different strategies and techniques in this book and integrate them into your lifestyle.

It's crucial for you to be patient with yourself along this journey, as it will take you some consistent time and effort to see the biohacking results you truly desire. When you realize that biohacking practices don't provide immediate results, you'll have more realistic expectations, which can make it easier to stick to this lifestyle change.

Biohacks Are the Same for Everyone

Everybody is different, which means that everyone's bodies will react to various biohacks differently. It's so important to consider this before you get started with this journey. Realizing that your body is unique will help you to practice biohacks specifically for your body. You practice trial and error, discovering a routine that works best for your mind and body.

This is why biohacking is a methodology that requires more thought and adaptation as you practice it. You need to discover the biology of your body and the specific biological potential you have. All of this personalized information will allow you to pick and choose the right biohacks, as well as implement them in a way that is most suited for your biological makeup.

All Biohacking Methods Are Supported by Science

Though biohacking is a scientifically-researched methodology, not every method is supported by science. Some techniques are experimental, and others are purely used based on other people's experiences. It's important to know when a biohack is scientifically proven, or whether it's an experiment or personal. Just because it may not be supported by science doesn't make it unsafe or invalid, as many biohackers have received positive results from it.

Real-Life Success Stories

You are more than capable of adapting your lifestyle to biohacking. Once you realize this, you'll be able to unlock all of your untapped potential. Biohacking may be just what you need to make the transformation in your life that you've been longing for. Let these success stories inspire you to integrate biohacking into your lifestyle:

- **Rich Lee.** Rich Lee's journey with biohacking has been focused on integrating technology with his biology. He has practiced some of the most extreme body modifications. With magnets and chips in his fingers, he's able to program himself to link to websites and perform other amazing tasks. A chip in his forearm constantly monitors his temperature. These technological advances have provided him with convenience and health in his life.

- **Corina Ingram-Noehr.** Corina's biohacking routine is more intense than many biohackers out there. Her daily ritual entails a combination of technological practices and strict diets. She is known to take up to 20 vitamins every day. She practices cold therapy and ensures that she boosts her immunity by wearing shorts in the coldest temperatures.

Though these are some extreme biohackers, they still reap the benefits from this practice. Biohacking may seem challenging to accomplish and you may even be hesitant about how beneficial and life-changing these biohacks can actually be for you. Reading these success stories of some of the most expert biohackers should make you feel motivated for the potential you can release with biohacking.

Chapter 2:

Biohacking for Optimal Nutrition

What you fuel your body with makes a big impact on how it feels and functions. When you're exploring the world of biohacking, you'll discover how connected your mind and gut truly are. Making this connection thrive with optimal nutrition will improve the way you feel, and it will accelerate the progress you make along this journey!

You'll be able to reach all of your greatest physical and health goals when you're mindful of the foods you fuel your body with. Revolutionizing your diet is the first step to transforming your life with biohacking.

The Role of Nutrition in Biohacking

When you consider nutrition and biohacking, you may just think about being healthy, but when it comes to considering these crucial ways of life together, we need to dive deeper into nutrition and what it means to you and your overall well-being. Nutrition is vital if you want to be healthy, but it's even more important to consider when you're practicing biohacking.

As you submerge yourself in the experience of biohacking, you're working toward exploring the most biologically advanced version of yourself. In order to achieve these biological advancements and your full potential, you need to be fueling your body with the right foods.

The Importance of Gut Health

Your gut is known to be the second mind, as it influences how you think and feel each day. When your gut is not doing well, you may find that you are more emotionally distressed, cognitively distracted, and physically overwhelmed. If you want to unleash the best, healthiest version of yourself, you need to ensure that your gut health is in top shape. If you're still unsure of what makes gut health so important, these are some reasons why it's so important:

- **Absorbing all of the nutrients in your body.** Having great gut health allows all of the nutrients in your diet to absorb into your bloodstream. This can ultimately allow you to digest your food better, as well as having smooth and efficient bowel movements. With good gut health, you're finally able to reap all of the benefits from the nutritional foods that you consume.

- **Boosting your immune system.** When you prioritize your gut health, you will find that you get sick less often. Not only do you experience fewer stomach issues, but you also find yourself feeling healthier and ready to take on everyday life. Being sick less often can help you to improve your physical performance, as well as help you to live a longer and healthier life.

- **Improving mental health.** Your gut health can have a huge impact on your mental space and how you're doing emotionally. If you want to boost your overall mental health, you need to start looking at how you nourish your gut. You become less stressed and upset, as you're able to tackle your stressors and issues. Our guts and emotions are so strongly linked, so when you look after your gut health, your emotions will feel more stable.

With all of this being said, how do you go about ensuring that your gut health is prioritized? Through biohacking, you'll be able to change your eating habits to ensure your gut health, as well as your overall health. You'll learn to nourish your body with the right foods and nutrients to help you gain strength, health, and biological brilliance.

Revolutionize Your Diet

Before you completely transform your diet, it's valuable for you to take some time to consider what your current diet looks like. What are some of the main food groups or food items that you often indulge in? How healthy would you say your diet currently is, and do you put much thought and effort into the meals you make and eat? Answering all of these questions will allow you to fully revolutionize your diet in a way that helps you to thrive more.

Developing Healthy Eating Habits

The best way for you to revolutionize your diet is by introducing yourself to healthy habits that improve what you consume in your daily life. It's all about integrating these habits into your daily routine until they are a healthy way of life for you. These are a few healthy habits you should consider integrating into your day-to-day life:

- **Being more mindful as you eat.** When you have a very chaotic life, it can be easy to find yourself caught up in the stress of life, which can result in you developing unhealthy eating habits. You eat your meals on the go, skip meals when you're busy, and eat the wrong foods that aren't good for you. You may end up eating too much or too little, as you're not being mindful of the food you put into your body. It's time for you to eat with more mindfulness, which means that you're observant and aware of the foods that you consume. Doing this will ensure that you are eating the right foods that align with the diet you've set for yourself.

- **Drinking more water.** It's so crucial to drink sufficient water each day. Though you may think that you drink enough water every day, it can be easy to go through day-to-day life without drinking at least two liters of water. If you find yourself struggling to get through your required amount of water each day, you will find that it has a negative toll on your overall health and well-being, which can be seen through physical and mental symptoms. It's so important to make a habit of drinking lots of water each day, and you can accomplish this by developing useful habits. For example, you can drink a glass of water with each meal you eat, or you can carry around a large two-liter bottle of water that you ensure you finish every day.

- **Introduce the right foods into your diet.** Of course, one of the most crucial ways for you to live a healthier life is by introducing yourself to the right foods that will make your body happy. Eating the right foods that help your body to thrive will provide you with the nutrients you may need to biohack your body to its full potential. Learning which foods are processed, high in sugar and bad for you, will help you to discover what type of foods with the right nutrients you should be looking for.

As you learn about the diets you can explore, the nutrients you must consume, and ways you can personalize a diet for your health and well-being, these healthy eating habits should be kept in consideration. If you're eating mindfully, drinking enough water, and introducing the right foods into your daily diet, you will have no problem biohacking your diet.

How to Change Your Diet

When you're so used to eating in a certain way, it can be challenging to completely transform your diet. You're so used to your eating habits that it can feel impossible to let go of these eating habits. These following tips can help you to change your diet more efficiently:

- **Start with small changes.** If changing your diet altogether seems a bit overwhelming, you should start off with smaller changes and work toward fully transforming your entire diet. When you change your eating habits one at a time, it can feel a lot more manageable for you. Start by cutting out that soda that you drink every day and slowly progress to more changes. The more changes you make, the easier it will be for you to completely transform your diet. Small changes will be the start of your grand journey.

- **Keep yourself accountable.** If you truly want to see results with your new diet, you need to be keeping yourself accountable regularly. You're the only person who is in charge of what you consume every day. Even if you find yourself frequently surrounded by temptations, you should be strict with yourself and make the decisions that you know are better for you in the long run.

- **Be patient.** With any change you make to your lifestyle or your everyday habits, you need to be patient with yourself. If you are too anxious for results and you don't give yourself the necessary time to see results, you may give up before you can even see what a fresh diet can do for you. Results don't come overnight when it comes to changing what you eat, so be patient with yourself and this process.

- **Treat yourself.** With all of this being said, you should still aim to treat yourself every once in a while in life. You deserve having your favorite foods, but in moderation. You can use treats as an incentive for when you make good progress with your healthy goals. Treating yourself seldom can also help you to reach your health and diet goals, as you find yourself satisfying your cravings, giving you the ability to remain strict and accountable with yourself. If you don't treat yourself every now and then, you may find yourself giving up on a diet, binging, or cheating on your diet frequently.

Changing your diet requires a lot of discipline and hard work. The more you work toward it, the easier it will start to become for you. Changing a diet is never easy, so it's important for you to be kind to yourself and avoid putting too much pressure on yourself. We will discuss some effective diets that you can practice shortly.

Biohacking Your Plate

Mindless eating is something we're all guilty of practicing every now and then. It can be so challenging to be mindful of what you put on your plate every day, especially when you have a busy schedule. This may result in you turning to fast and easy meals and filling your everyday plate with foods that don't leave you feeling satisfied and full.

Biohacking your plate is all about ensuring that you fill it with all of the nutrients you need for a healthy diet. As we explore what your plate should consist of, you should consider how to make this relative to the diets that you may explore. Regardless of what diet you're on, you want to ensure that every meal is balanced, nutritious, and healthy for you.

Knowing Your Macro and Micronutrients

Before we explore what a well-balanced meal should look like for you, you need to be more aware and mindful of macro and micronutrients. Knowing what they are and how they play an important role in your diet can help you to put together meals that satisfy and nourish you fully. Consuming the specific macro and micronutrients that you need plays a large role in your biohacking journey.

Macronutrients

Macronutrients are large food categories that are required for our bodies in large amounts. These categories make up the main three food groups, and it's crucial for you to ensure that you include them in each of your meals. The most significant three macronutrients are as follows:

- **Carbohydrates.** Carbohydrates are often viewed as evil in the diet culture, as people think they contribute to weight gain. However, carbohydrates are critical for your body's daily functioning. Complex carbohydrates help your digestion system by providing you with great fiber for your gut health and they keep you full for longer. They also provide you with both instant and stored energy. When you're looking for the right carbohydrates to consume, you should avoid processed, high-sugar carbohydrates, and consume complex carbs with nutritional value.

- **Protein.** When you consume protein, it's digested as amino acids. Out of 20 of the amino acids your body absorbs, nine of them are essential for your health and day-to-day functioning. These amino acids help to build and repair the proteins in your body. They provide structure to your organ's membranes, as well as create a healthy pH balance within your body. Consuming protein also contributes to the production and balance of enzymes and hormones in your body.

- **Fats.** Foods containing fats are broken down into fatty acids and glycerol when you consume them. These lipids or fats are needed in your body to fulfill a variety of functions such as storing energy and optimizing cell membrane health. Fatty acids are also crucial to improve the absorption of certain vitamins in your bloodstream. Fat is a great insulation for your organs.

A good healthy balanced meal has all three of these macronutrients included, as they make up the main food groups. If you want to maintain your body's structure and functioning, you need to consume the right amounts of each food group.

Micronutrients

Micronutrients are a much smaller category of foods, but they are just as important. These are the vitamins and minerals your body needs to function optimally. They provide a variety of functions in your body each day without you realizing it. Deficiencies in certain micronutrients can take a toll on your overall health, which can be displayed in negative symptoms like lethargy, health conditions, and a higher risk of catching diseases.

Your micronutrients include vitamins and minerals. There is a long list of vitamins that make up the micronutrients your body needs, these are just a few of the most important ones and their benefits:

- **Vitamin B.** When it comes to your B vitamins, there are a variety of different types you should be enriching your body with. They provide you with so many crucial benefits such as cell growth, energy levels, functions of your brain, nerve functions, and the growth of red blood cells.

- **Vitamin C.** Vitamin C is a crucial vitamin your body requires to remain healthy and boost your immune system, providing you with antioxidants.

- **Vitamin A.** This vitamin boosts your immunity, enhances your skin health, and improves your vision.

- **Vitamin D.** Vitamin D strengthens your bones, muscles, and your health.

- **Vitamin E.** To further improve your immune system or vision, you should add vitamin E to your diet.

- **Vitamin K.** Vitamin K can allow you to heal at a faster rate, as it promotes blood clotting and wound healing.

Minerals are just as important and necessary for your body as vitamins are. This is a list of some of the most crucial vitamins you should be putting in your body:

- **Magnesium.** Allowing your body to use glucose for energy.

- **Calcium.** Strengthening your bones and regulating your heart functioning.

- **Iodine.** Aiding the production of thyroid hormones.

- **Iron.** Helping to fulfill bodily functions such as the transportation of oxygen.

- **Zinc.** Boosting your growth development and bodily functions.

- **Potassium.** Valuable for the nervous system.

- **Sodium.** Promoting healthy blood circulation.

You receive micronutrients from the fruits and vegetables you consume every day. When you go grocery shopping, it's important for you to be on the lookout for fresh produce that contains all of the micronutrients your body needs.

What Should Your Plate Look Like?

Now that you know all about the macro and micronutrients your body requires, we can explore what your plate should look like. It's crucial to learn how to properly balance each plate you consume in a day so that you're providing yourself with all of the nutrients your body craves. 50% of your plate should consist of vegetables, 25% healthy protein, and 25% whole grains. Of course, not every meal has to look like this, but you should try to create balanced plates like this.

Designing a Biohacking Diet for Improved Energy, Focus, and Vitality

It's time for you to take control of your life and how you feel each day. Designing a biohacking diet for you will improve your gut health, which will strengthen the relationship with your mind and gut. A better diet will leave you filled with life, sharpened concentration, and overall improved health.

Elimination Diet

Did you know you could currently be eating foods that don't seem unhealthy, but they're actually taking a toll on your body? Because your gut is unique and functions in a specific way, there may be foods that you're intolerant to. When you adapt to a healthier diet, you find that you still aren't reaching the full potential you had hoped for. In this case, there may be foods unsuitable for you that you need to cut out. You just need to identify what these foods are!

The elimination diet is the most effective way for you to identify which foods are good for you and which ones disagree with your gut health. Through the process of trial and elimination, you discover how your body reacts to certain foods. Follow these steps to practice the elimination diet successfully:

1. **Write in a food journal.** Before you start changing your diet through elimination, you need to spend a few days recording the way you eat. Doing this can help you to discover your current eating patterns and the foods that you eat quite frequently. As you record in your food journal, it's so important for you to ensure that you're eating how you would normally eat, including both the good and bad. Write down every single food item you consume, as this will provide you with the most accurate results. We will discuss how to use a food journal in more ways further on in this book.

2. **Study your food journal.** Once you've recorded your consumption for each day, you should take the time to study this journal. Try and look for patterns or eating habits that you practice on a regular basis. Identify the foods that you eat really frequently, as these may be contributing to your gut health issues. In this journal, you should also have records of any stomach issues you've been having, so you can correlate the gut health issues with the foods you've eaten that aren't agreeing with you.

3. **Cut out common intolerances.** Now that you've done all of this research on yourself, you can start the elimination process. It's important for you to eliminate foods that you're most likely intolerant to. To do this, you need to consider some of the most common intolerances that your gut may be sensitive to. Some common foods that people are usually intolerant to are dairy, gluten, and caffeine. Spend a week cutting out dairy first, then see how you feel afterward. Now practice the same elimination techniques with gluten and then caffeine. If you don't notice any change, you can try an elimination diet with some less common intolerances like salicylates, a chemical released by certain plants that you can find in various fruits,

28

vegetables, and spices. Amines are another intolerance that includes tyramine, serotonin, and histamine, which can be found in certain fruits, vegetables, alcohol, and mature foods. Lastly, fructose is a rare food intolerance which is a natural sugar that can be found in fruits, fruit juices, and honey.

4. **Cut out the most common foods in your diet.** If you cut out common intolerances and you aren't noticing a change in your gut health, you should go back to the drawing board and identify all of the foods that you eat the most. Looking for these patterns in your everyday life will help you to identify the best foods for you to eliminate from your diet. Even if these foods are some of your favorite foods, you should try the elimination method, as you never know what foods could alter your moods, energy levels, and overall gut health.

5. **Adjust your diet.** Now that you've done all of this research and elimination, you have a better picture of what foods you need to cut out of your diet. Knowing this information can help you to adjust your diet successfully. Now you know which foods aren't agreeing with you, so you can ensure that you're replacing them with better foods for your body. For example, if you're lactose intolerant, you can avoid drinking cow's milk by replacing it with almond milk, oat milk, or soy milk. Finding the right replacements for the foods you're intolerant to will leave your stomach happy without having to compromise the foods you love.

As you go through these steps, it's valuable for you to record all of the information you gather. Doing this will help you to feel more in control of this process, as you have all of your recorded information easily accessible. It can also help you when you want to go back and adjust.

Intermittent Fasting

Another form of diet that is valuable for you to explore is intermittent fasting. It's the process of training your body via specific eating intervals. Intermittent fasting can be explored in a variety of ways, depending on what works best for you and your body. You can either not eat during a certain period of the day or a specific period of the week.

Practicing intermittent fasting can be quite beneficial for you if you're looking to reach specific biological goals. Some benefits of this diet include reduced inflammation, anti-aging properties, a boost in brain health, and it can also speed up your metabolism. These are a few intermittent fasting methods you can explore:

- **The 16:8 method.** This fasting method is for when you choose an eight-hour period each day to eat and you fast for the other 16 hours of the day. If you choose this form of fasting, it's advised for you to pick eight hours of your day when you're usually the hungriest and need food as a source of energy. For example, if you're someone who doesn't eat breakfast, but you're really hungry in the afternoon and evening, you can make your eight hours 12 p.m.–8 p.m.

- **The 5:2 diet.** The premise of this method is that you eat normally five days of the week, by maintaining your regular calorie intake, but on two days of the week, you eat considerably less, between 500 and 600 calories. For example, if your normal day-to-day calorie intake is 1,900 calories, you choose five days of the week when you need the most energy to consume these calories. Then for two days of the week where you're less busy and less physically active, you consume between 500 and 600 calories. To successfully practice this method, you must eat fewer meals, eat foods low in calories, and ensure that you're keeping note of the calories in each food item you consume.

- **Eat-stop-eat.** This intermittent fasting method is a bit stricter, as you have to go a full 24 hours without eating anything. During the week you eat normally, but you choose one or even two days a week where you eat absolutely nothing for 24 hours. All you can consume is water on these fasting days. If you choose two days a week, be sure to set them far apart. You should only choose to fast on days when you know you'll be less active and you don't require lots of energy; otherwise, you could risk hurting yourself.

When you're choosing an intermittent fasting method for you, it's crucial to discover what's most sustainable for you. Try out each method and determine what fits into your lifestyle and eating habits. One of the most popular, convenient, and sustainable diets for many is the 16:8 method.

Practicing intermittent fasting can help you achieve lots of the physical and mental goals you've set for yourself on this journey. You can boost your cognitive capabilities, balance your hormones, and reduce inflammation. You will even be able to reach specific body goals that you've been trying to achieve for a long time.

Ketogenic Diet

A ketogenic diet, also commonly known as a keto diet, is a diet that consists of less carbohydrates and more fats. When you reduce the amount of carbohydrates you consume, it causes your body to go into a metabolic state of ketosis. This form of diet helps you to burn fat for energy, as well as lowering your blood sugar levels. It can be challenging to adapt to this diet, as you are introducing yourself to different food habits, so these are some tips that will help you to adjust to a ketogenic diet:

- **Know what to eat and what not to eat.** Keto is all about knowing which carb-filled foods you need to avoid, and which healthy fats you should start including in your diet. You should avoid sugary and processed foods, grains, or starches. When you're introducing more fats to your diet, it's important to avoid unhealthy fats and focus on enriching and nutrient-dense fats like fatty fish, eggs, meat, cheese, nuts, healthy oils, avocado, and low-carb vegetables.

- **Plan your meals efficiently.** Practicing a keto diet successfully is all about knowing how to plan each meal efficiently, ensuring that they are balanced with the right nutrients. A great example of a successful day of eating keto includes a breakfast consisting of a spinach omelet with tomatoes, chicken salad for lunch, and a dinner made of squash for spaghetti with a bolognese sauce. If you do plan on having carbohydrates in your meal, ensure that it makes up a very small percentage of your plate.

- **Explore various ketogenic diets.** Within the ketogenic diet, there are specific forms of this diet that you can explore. Your standard keto diet is the most popular. This diet consists of 70% fat, 20% protein, and 10% carbohydrates. In a cyclical ketogenic diet, you choose five days of the week to follow a low-carb diet, but for two days of the week, you eat higher-carb meals. For the days when you heat more carbs, consider doing more exercise. You can also explore high protein keto, which is similar to regular keto, but instead, you're consuming more protein and a little less of carbs and fat.

There are various benefits you can receive from practicing a keto diet, as it is a great meal plan for individuals with diabetes, as well as being really effective for weight loss. Keto can reduce your risk of heart disease and cancer. It can also improve any symptoms you may be experiencing from Alzheimer's disease, epilepsy, and polycystic ovary syndrome.

Paleo Diet

The paleo diet allows you to adapt to the expected eating habits of the Paleolithic Era. This era dates between 2.5 million and 10,000 years ago, and the diet is known to consist of vegetables, fruits, lean meat, nuts, fish, eggs, and seeds. This diet can be seen as very similar to keto, as the amount of carbs you consume for both diets is very limited. However, these diets differ as keto is a diet focused on fats, whereas paleo is a more equally balanced diet, excluding carbohydrates.

Though there are certain things you should and shouldn't consume for this form of diet, practicing a paleo diet can be lenient, as you have a large variety of foods to choose from. It's all about cutting out processed foods and refined sugars while making both big and small changes within your food choices. Consuming lean and grass-fed meat, using oils from nuts and fruits like olive oil, and avoiding starchy vegetables like corn and potatoes. These are all valuable changes that will allow you to practice a paleo diet successfully.

Cut Out Processed Sugars

It can be challenging to find any food without processed sugars nowadays, as most tasty foods have processed additives that make them so addictive. If you want to transform your diet for the better, cutting out processed sugars is one of the best approaches for you to take. It can be so challenging to cut out sugar, as it is everywhere and impossible to avoid, as well as it's just so good to eat. Whichever diet you decide to follow, if you want to reach your biological potential, you must ensure that you cut out processed sugar. The following tips will help you to effectively cut sugar out of your diet in the best ways possible:

- **Read your labels.** Labels can tell you everything you need to know about what's in a certain product. We can often consume products that we just assume are healthy for us, but when we read the labels, we realize how many negative additives are truly in our foods. When you're reading the labels of the food in your pantry, consider giving away the food items that will not be fitting for your new biohacking lifestyle. When going shopping, focus on buying foods that have compatible labels that will provide you with food of great nutritional value.

- **Making healthy replacements.** After reading the labels of the food you buy next and the food that is currently in your pantry, it's important for you to make the necessary replacements. Cutting sugar from your diet doesn't mean cutting a lot of food from your daily consumption, as you can make healthy replacements that keep you full and satisfied. If you're craving something sweet, eat some healthy fruits. Maybe you'd really like some processed and saturated fats, so you can have a healthier snack like popcorn. Consuming healthier replacements for your favorite unhealthy food will keep you more committed and disciplined to your change in diet.

- **Detox your diet.** Nowadays, you can find sugar in almost everything that you eat. We can indulge in some of our favorite snacks or meals without realizing the processed sugars or saturated fats that are included in the ingredients. It's time for you to go through a few weeks where you completely detox and cut out the sugars that aren't good for you. Doing this may be tricky at first, as you find your body craving the sugars that aren't good for you. However, being strict with yourself and your detox period will result in you receiving the best long-term results, as you will be able to adjust to a lifestyle of consuming less sugar. If you want to go the extra mile with your detox, you can prioritize consuming liquids with nutritional value, instead of consuming solid foods, as this can help you to reset your gut entirely.

Consuming less sugar will improve your health drastically and make your gut really happy. You'll also find that consuming less sugar improves your energy levels. There is a common misconception that sugar boosts your energy, but in reality, sugar has the opposite effect. When you consume sugar, you will receive an initial boost in your energy, but as time passes you will start to crash.

Let Go of Toxic Consumption

To follow up on the previous tip, you should avoid all forms of toxic consumption, as this could be taking a toll on your gut health. These unhealthy habits can be so easy to practice, as they provide us with a sense of comfort, but if you want to reach your physical potential and live the best long and healthy life possible, you need to let go of these toxic consumption habits:

- **Fast food.** When you're feeling too lazy to cook and you're craving some deep fried, greasy, and unhealthy food, fast food may be your first resort. It can be such a comfort to indulge in fast food, even though we know that it's not good for us. It's time to cut the habit of turning to fast food whenever you're feeling down or lazy, as it's these frequent unhealthy meals that are stopping you from getting your health goals back.

- **Smoking.** If you're someone who struggles with intense stress, you may use smoking as a negative coping mechanism. It relieves you of stress for a few seconds, but you find yourself needing to smoke one cigarette after another trying to chase that feeling of relief. Smoking cigarettes can have a huge negative impact on your well-being and longevity, as you are at high risk for respiratory diseases such as lung cancer.

- **Alcohol.** Though there's nothing wrong with having a glass of wine every now and then, making a habit out of drinking alcohol every day can take a toll on your body. Becoming addicted to alcohol can be really easy when you're overwhelmed with life, so letting go of a habit that seems simple can feel almost impossible. Being addicted to alcohol is a serious issue you shouldn't take lightly. Seek professional help when necessary. Consuming alcohol every day can negatively affect your physical health, as it puts you at high risk for certain diseases in the future.

Ensuring that you let go of these toxic habits will help your biohacking journey become more successful. Though it can be easier said than done to let go of these habits, it's important for you to make the habit each day to let go of this routine. Start off with baby steps and warm your way up to cutting these habits out of your routine entirely. If you find that these toxic habits are really taking a toll on your body, you need to seek professional help.

Strategies for Personalizing Your Nutrition Plan and Optimizing Nutrient Absorption

You now know some effective and practical ways to transform your diet for the better. Not every diet will be effective for everyone, as you will experience various outcomes from different eating styles. What's important is that you make the effort to try out different diets that may be most suitable for you.

Try Different Diets

If you want to find the diet that is best for you, you need to try out a variety of diets. Only once you've explored these various food changes, will you be able to have a better idea of what is most suitable for you and your body. Even if you think that a specific diet won't work for you, take the opportunity to try it out anyway, as you never know how effective it may be.

It's important for you to give each of these diets a proper try before switching to new ones. You need to be on each diet for long enough for you to see real results. From this, you'll be able to make a decision based on all the information you've collected. Using a food journal will help you to track the results of each diet so you know which one will work best for you.

Something that's valuable to remember is that your body adapts and grows with time. This means that you'll need to try out different diets and daily meals with time. Your body may require a different variety of nutrients as you grow. It's crucial not to stick to one diet forever, as this may decrease the quality of results you receive.

Make Use of a Food Journal

As we've briefly discussed earlier, a food journal is a great and effective way for you to take control of your eating habits and revolutionize your diet. A food journal may be just what you need to track and process the food you're eating so that you can reach your goals. Using a food journal is quite simple, but you want to ensure that you're using it in the most effective ways. These are some crucial tips you should consider:

- **Keep your journal with you 24/7.** If you want to experience the best results from your journal, you need to ensure that you are logging everything that you consume each day. You can't just keep it at home because you never know when you might be eating when you leave the house. If you only track what you eat at home, you'll leave out a large portion of your diet. Ensure you use a book or journal you can carry around with you always.

- **Write down every detail.** It's so important to ensure that you are including every single detail in your food journal, as this is the only way that you will achieve accurate results. You may just write down the general meals that you eat, but you should include each and every detail of these foods, as well as the ingredients you used to prepare these meals.

- **Record gut health issues.** To be even more specific and accurate with your food journal, you should record any of the gut health issues you may be experiencing. Be really specific and record the exact day and time you experience these struggles. Doing this will help you to realize what foods may be disagreeing with you, as well as help you make the necessary changes to your diet.

- **Track your progress.** The greatest benefit of having a food journal is that you're able to track your progress and discover how far you've come with your journey. This can not only impress you, as you notice how far you've come, but it will also help you to identify what's working with your diets, and what's not working. From this, you'll be able to make the changes in your diet that you need.

Your food journal should be your go to tool that you use to achieve your diet transformation. It may seem challenging to continuously record in this journal, especially when you're really busy, but the more you do it, the easier it will become for you. Soon you'll be writing in your food journal without even thinking about it first.

Chapter 3:

Mastering Sleep and Recovery

Getting sufficient sleep every night will give you the mental and physical strength you need to become the best version of yourself. Lacking sufficient sleep can have a variety of negative impacts on you, as you find yourself frustrated and irritable. Looking after yourself through high quality sleep and recovery will provide you with a sense of bliss and fulfillment that encourages you to grow. When you optimize your sleep schedule every night, you'll have the energy and ability to achieve all of your goals.

The Importance of Sufficient Sleep

When we think about our health, we can often focus on the foods we eat, our physical fitness level, or our mental agility. We usually overlook our need for sleep, as it can feel like there are never enough hours within a day to get everything you need done. This can result in you compromising sleep to prioritize other tasks in your life. It's time to make sleep one of your biggest priorities, as getting sufficient sleep is so important for the following reasons:

- **Improves concentration and focus.** If you're someone who really struggles to stay focused during important tasks, it may be a sign that your body is craving more sleep. When you've had a bad night's sleep or you've pulled an all-nighter to complete an important task, you will find it almost impossible to focus on the next day. The more important the task or responsibility is, the more challenging it will be for you to stay focused and productive. Sleeping sufficiently each night will allow you to tackle your work with focus and intent each day.

- **Maximizes your athletic performance.** If you're currently focused on becoming the best athlete you can be, sufficient sleep will allow you to achieve optimal athletic performance. Your body requires enough sleep to build muscles and recover. Sufficient sleep can also enhance motor skills, muscular capabilities, and reaction times, which can all contribute to maximizing your athletic performance. Getting sufficient sleep can also prevent you from being at risk of injuries when you're practicing sports or athletic activities regularly. This will allow you to push your athletic limits without worrying about hurting yourself. Injuries can interrupt the progress you make when trying to unlock your full athletic biological potential.

- **Boosts your immune system.** When you find yourself falling ill more frequently, it may be a sign that you need more rest to boost your immune system. Sleeping sufficiently every night will boost your immunity drastically. You'll find yourself getting sick less, which can help you to reach your full biological potential. If you do get sick, you're able to heal and recover at a faster rate.

- **Enhancing your emotional well-being.** Getting an insufficient amount of sleep can take a negative toll on you emotionally. You find yourself getting more overwhelmed than you usually would, as you're short-tempered, more sensitive, and easily frustrated. Obstacles, negative comments, and unwanted circumstances can be a lot more overwhelming to handle than they usually are for you. You feel a lot more stable and prepared to tackle any issues that may be coming your way in life.

- **Provides patience for biohacking.** Lastly, and certainly not least, sleeping a sufficient number of hours each night can provide you with the patience you need to tackle your biohacking strategies and techniques. You feel more prepared to achieve all of the specific routines that are required of you, which allows you to be consistent with biohacking. This will provide you with the best long-term results.

Sleep is so crucial for our advancement in life. If you want to transform into the best version of yourself, you need to be giving your body the sufficient rest it needs to recover and grow. When you ensure your body gets sufficient sleep every night, you will find yourself able to achieve a lot more along this journey.

Why Recovery Is Crucial for Biohacking

Nurturing your body is just as important as practicing discipline. When you look after yourself through recovery, you will find yourself more productive than ever! We all deserve some TLC, especially when it's in the form of self-care. Recovering will give you the strength you need to embrace biohacking to the fullest! These are some ways you can practice recovery:

- **Preventing muscle injuries.** When you give yourself time to recover, you're less likely to experience any injuries as you push yourself physically. If you aren't recovering, stretching, or looking after your body, you may find that when you participate in physical activities, you're a lot more likely to injure yourself. Injuring yourself will prevent you from achieving the progress you want for yourself physically.

- **Creating longevity.** Biohacking is all about seeking long-term results and success, instead of prioritizing short-term growth. If you keep pushing yourself without taking breaks or precautions, you may see fast results, but you will find yourself burning out, getting injured, or giving up from exhaustion. Taking necessary recovery measures allows you to achieve long-term results that make your present and future life easier and more enjoyable.

- **An act of self-care.** Prioritizing recovery shows that you have a sense of love and self-care for your body. Sometimes, it's important to show ourselves the compassion and care we have for our bodies and overall health. Showing how much you truly care about yourself and your well-being will help you to be more committed to biohacking, as treating yourself to self-care allows you to become the best version of yourself.

If you want to reach peak physical and athletic performance, you need to be open to spending a sufficient amount of time recovering your mind and body. Recovery will be the best thing you can do for yourself as you embrace biohacking. Remember that as much as pushing yourself beyond your limits and getting out of your comfort zone will help you to grow, resting and recovering will also provide you with the strength you need to achieve self-improvement.

Biohacking Sleep

Now that you know how crucial sleep is for you to achieve your full potential throughout this journey, it's important to learn how you can improve the amount, quality, and efficiency of your sleep through biohacking. Finding helpful hacks and routines can allow you to develop a nighttime routine that prioritizes efficient and peaceful sleep every night.

Biohacking Insomnia

If you try to get sufficient hours of sleep every night, but you find that your insomnia is holding you back, biohacking can help you to relieve yourself of this tedious struggle. Having insomnia every night can be extremely frustrating, as you find yourself really wanting to have better sleep, but no matter how hard you try, your insomnia prevents you from getting the rest you so deeply desire. Try out these tips to cure your insomnia with biohacking:

- **Reduce blue light.** A modern problem many of us face is too much exposure to blue light before sleeping. How often do you find yourself scrolling on your phone before going to sleep at night? You get caught up in videos and once you find yourself getting drowsy, you put your phone down. However, as you get ready to sleep you feel more awake than ever.

- **Use supplements.** There are certain natural and perfectly innovative supplements that can help you to fall asleep throughout the night. Finding the right supplements to consume before sleeping will allow you to be more tranquil and relaxed, which causes you to experience deep sleep. We will discuss supplements in more detail further on in this book, so you can discover which supplements you should explore and how.

- **Prioritize your gut health.** If you work on prioritizing your gut health by revolutionizing your diet for the better, you will find that it actually helps you sleep better at night. Knowing which foods you should eat at night and which ones you should avoid will ensure that you're consuming the right foods for optimal sleep.

- **Hack your sleeping patterns.** Being able to fix your sleeping patterns will help you to sleep more efficiently through the night. Developing an exact sleeping pattern will help you to develop some structure in your nighttime routine. Finding a time period that's best for you will allow your body to adapt to a strict cycle that you follow every night.

- **Polyphasic sleep patterns.** If you feel as though the traditional sleep schedule isn't working for you, you may find it valuable to try a polyphasic sleep schedule. This is when you sleep for more than two separate intervals in the day and night, instead of getting seven to nine hours of uninterrupted sleep at night. The benefits of following this sleeping schedule include experiencing less fatigue, being more productive throughout your day, and bettering your memory. You can follow a variety of schedules such as the Dymaxion schedule which entails having 30-minute nap intervals every six hours. Alternatively, you could try the Uberman schedule where you have 20-minute naps every four hours. When trying this schedule, play around with different intervals and time frames to see what works best for you, your daily schedule, and your body's health.

When you successfully manage to hack your sleeping schedule, you'll be able to reach the goals that you've been wanting to achieve. You become more alert, capable, and you achieve a sense of calm you didn't know was possible for you.

Hacking Your Circadian Rhythm

Your circadian rhythm is your sleep-wake routine throughout the 24 hours of each day. When your brain receives signals or cues such as lightness and darkness from your environment, it releases certain hormones and functions within your body that either influence wakefulness or sleepiness. If you want to achieve the best sleep each night and have more alertness during the day, it's imperative to hack your circadian rhythm. These are some effective ways you can accomplish it:

- **Understanding how it works.** Before you figure out how to hack your circadian rhythm, it's important to understand how your internal clock works. Your hormones and body cells contribute greatly to your circadian rhythm. Melatonin and cortisol are some of the main hormones that can make or break your internal sleep schedule. Melatonin is a hormone that influences the timing of your sleep schedule in response to darkness and external settings. Cortisol is a stress hormone that can negatively disrupt your circadian rhythm. Your body temperature also has a role in your circadian rhythm, as your temperature drops when you sleep and rises when you're awake.

- **Knowing what factors impact your circadian rhythm.** You could be practicing day-to-day tasks or habits that interfere with your circadian rhythm. This is why it's so valuable for you to know which factors can both positively and negatively influence this internal rhythm. If you're a night-shift worker, you'll find that your circadian rhythm is completely out of balance. You're used to being awake at night during the darkness, and you try to sleep during light hours. It is really challenging for your hormones to adjust to an unnatural schedule. If you have a lifestyle or work schedule that requires you to wake up at early hours in the morning, you may also struggle to achieve a healthy internal clock. Other factors that can impact you include stress, mental health conditions, certain medications, and unhealthy sleeping patterns like consuming caffeine in the evening.

- **Resetting your circadian rhythm.** To hack your circadian rhythm, you need to be able to adhere to a routine that works with your body. Choose a time frame that suits your schedule, as well as your body's natural fatigue. Considering your environment when sleeping is crucial to reset your internal clock, as you should ensure that your room isn't receiving any external light by investing in some blackout curtains (this can be really valuable if you're a night shift worker, as it can trick your brain into thinking it's nighttime, allowing you to achieve deeper sleep). If possible, regulating the temperature of your environment by making it cooler, can influence your body to release melatonin and enter a sleep state. To regulate your internal clock, it's valuable for you to expose yourself to more light during your waking hours. Spending more time outdoors can not only make you feel more awake, but it will also allow your circadian rhythm to become more responsive to light. Challenge yourself to exercise outdoors every day and you will find your internal clock successfully adjusting to this new schedule.

Once you reset your circadian rhythm, you'll feel more rested during your waking hours, and you'll experience deeper and more satisfying sleep. Having good quality sleep every day will give you the energy you need to conquer your new healthy biohacking lifestyle!

Biohacking Devices and Resources to Use

It's valuable for you to be open to various devices and resources that can allow you to achieve optimal sleep. Investing in these items can help you to tackle insomnia or any sleeping problems that may be holding you back in your journey. If there are devices and tools that can improve your quality and duration of sleep, why not try them out? Here are some great products to try:

- **Smart sleeping pad.** A sleeping pad is a device you place in or under your pillow which is linked via Bluetooth to your phone. You can use different settings to experience different benefits from your sleeping pad. It releases natural compounds like melatonin, which is a hormone that helps you to regulate your sleep, without you having to physically consume it.

- **Blinks sleep mask.** Using a sleep mask can be really effective for you to fall asleep, as it blocks out any of the light that keeps you awake. Its comfortable design makes your face feel comforted and relaxed. Its ability to block out blue light helps you to sleep through the night without distractions.

- **Diffuser.** Having a diffuser in your room is great for a number of reasons, especially when you're sleeping. You can use essential oils that promote relaxation and deeper sleep. We will discuss how this works with aromatherapy further on in this book.

Biohacking devices can make your sleeping experience a lot more peaceful and enjoyable. When you're constantly on the go, you have a lot of stress on your mind, and you put a lot of pressure on yourself, which can make it impossible to fall asleep and stay asleep. Use these devices to achieve deep sleep so that you have the strength and energy to get through each day with ease.

Practical Tips for Enhancing Recovery and Physical Performance

We've discussed how important it is to ensure that you prioritize recovery along this journey, as recovery ensures that you are reaching the best physical performance possible. You may find that when you push yourself, it takes a long time for your body to recover physically. Utilizing these practical tips can help you to enhance and improve your recovery time, which allows you to provide a better physical performance.

Prioritizing Muscle Recovery

If you want to achieve grand physical abilities, you need to be able to prioritize muscle recovery. When you're continuously putting your muscles under strain by doing extensive and intense physical activity, you'll find yourself experiencing a lot more aches and pains than you're used to.

If you're not taking the necessary precautions and measures when exercising, you will find that this pain becomes unbearable, which prevents you from pushing yourself past your limits. This is why it's so important for you to prioritize muscle recovery every time you plan on engaging in physical activity:

- **Warm-ups and cooldowns.** Before you exercise each day, it's crucial for you to practice your warm-ups. Doing this with each exercise will ensure that your muscles and tendons don't experience any aches and pains from your physical activity. Warming up before physical activity is crucial as you get your muscles loosened up and your blood flowing. Some examples of warm-ups include dynamic stretches, walking up and down stairs, and lunges and squats. It's important to warm up the specific muscles you're about to work out.

- **Cooldowns.** Cooldowns are necessary to boost and improve the recovery process. When you're training your body to the best of your abilities, you need to practice cooldowns to ensure that you achieve endurance. This allows you to achieve long-term physical performance, instead of receiving short-term results. Some forms of cooldowns you can explore are light jogging or walking, low intensity yoga, and body stretches and shake offs.

- **Listen to your body.** Though your biohacking journey should be all about pushing your body past its limits, you shouldn't push beyond what you're capable of. Exploring a biohacking journey is all about becoming the best version of yourself while listening to your body and what it needs. When you listen to your body and its needs, you're able to take breaks when necessary and push yourself within your limits.

When you put more effort into prioritizing your muscle recovery, you discover how beneficial it will be for your physical performance capabilities. You'll be able to achieve more from your biohacking journey when you allow your muscles to recover, grow, and strengthen. Look after your body so that it can look after you!

Nourish Your Body

When you want to integrate biohacking techniques and strategies into your everyday life, it's important for you to consider it holistically. You can't achieve peak physical performance if you aren't mindful of how you're nourishing your body. You also won't be able to achieve your fitness goals when you aren't resting or hydrating your body as much as you should be.

Realizing the importance of nourishing your body will allow you to treat and condition it in a way that results in optimal strength and recovery. When you're more physically active than you usually are, you need to ensure that you're eating the right foods with great dietary fiber and nutrients so that you have sufficient energy to successfully perform each exercise. You also want to ensure that you're including the macro and micronutrients that make you stronger, more capable, and fitter.

It's important to remember that when you're more physically active, your body requires more water to stay hydrated. You'll be sweating a lot more than you usually do, which requires you to drink more water so that you can replenish all of the water you've lost. Hydrating yourself will allow you to practice physical activity safely and productively. Always nourish yourself with the necessary nutrients to perform physical activities at your peak capabilities.

Have Rest Days

If you want to achieve ambitious physical goals, you may find yourself wanting to practice a new physical activity each day. Though it's valuable to diversify the types of fitness activities and practices you use, it's important for you to have rest days every week. These rest days are what help your body to recover from strenuous activity so that you can achieve the best physical performance. If you want to learn how to plan rest days effectively without negatively impacting your progress, consider the following tips:

- **Choosing one or two days in your week.** If you want to receive optimal rest days for your mind and body, you should aim for at least one or two days per week to rest. Two days is best, but one day of complete rest can be sufficient. On these rest days, ensure that you refrain from physical activity, and indulge in self-care. Treat your body with a nice soothing hot bath.

- **Active rest days.** If you don't want to take a complete day off, you can explore active rest days, which provide you with the same benefits while still stimulating yourself. Active rest days are when you are still moving your body with physical activity, but you aren't doing anything intense that might strain your muscles. For example, going for a walk or practicing low intensity yoga.

Investing your time into these rest days will help you to be more productive during your active days. You'll find that you're able to perform more, as you give your body enough time to recover and even build muscle mass. Taking rest days will also prevent you from experiencing injuries, as you give yourself enough time to heal.

Chapter 4:

Boosting Cognitive Abilities and Mental Performance

Being able to optimize your cognitive ability can be the best advancement you do for yourself and your professional life. Boosting your cognitive abilities can provide you with pride and joy, as you're able to accomplish things you never knew you could. Your brain is capable of so much, so it's time for you to give yourself the opportunity to discover what your best mental performance could look like!

Throughout this chapter, we will explore specific biohacking practices that can enhance your mental performance and cognitive abilities. Enhancing your cognitive functions through supplements, cutting-edge technology, a healthy lifestyle, and nootropics will provide you with the results you desire.

Nootropics may be a new term for many, but as a biohacker exploring this natural enhancer is a must, as they boost your mental performance. We will explain everything you need to know about nootropics shortly.

Biohacking the Brain for Improved Cognitive Function

If you've always been a more athletic and physically fit individual, you may have moments when you think that you lack cognitive skills. You underestimate your intelligence and everything that you could achieve mentally because you're yet to reach your full cognitive potential. When you practice biohacking for the brain, you'll realize that you're capable of so much more cognitively.

Understanding the Brain Structure and How it Functions

The brain structure is very complex, but understanding the basics of how it's structured and how it functions will help you to understand how you can biohack your cognitive abilities. Our brains control our every movement and bodily function, which is why it's so valuable to know how to use it to your advantage. The brain is made up of many parts, but the three main parts include the following:

- **Cerebrum.** The cerebrum is the biggest part of your brain, making up 80% of your brain. It contains all of the lobes, which are sections of the brain that fulfill different functions. It allows you to experience the five senses of sight, sound, smell, touch, and taste, as well as to regulate and process your learning, emotions, and reasoning.

- **Cerebellum.** The cerebellum is situated at the back of your brain. It provides you with the function of staying balanced, keeping your posture, and allowing you to stay coordinated. It has special sensors that can identify your movements or shifts in balance, sending signals to keep you balanced and coordinated. This part of your brain is also exercised when you're practicing your motor skills.

- **Brain stem.** Located at the bottom lower section of your brain is your brain stem. The brain stem connects to the rest of your body via the spinal cord. It is used to regulate your body's automatic functions such as breathing, sleeping, blinking, and heart rate. These crucial actions aren't practiced consciously, as your brain stem sends signals through your spinal cord to fulfill these necessary bodily functions.

These three parts work together to help your body function efficiently on a day-to-day basis. It's important to fulfill a healthy lifestyle and practice the biohacking tips in this chapter to ensure that you optimize the functioning of your brain.

Diet to Fulfill Your Nutritional Needs

Your diet is the most important component of biohacking for your cognitive functioning. We've discussed how you should enrich and nourish your diet with the right foods for your well-being, but now we'll discuss some specific diet changes you can make to boost your cognitive skills.

It's so important to ensure that you add the right foods to your diet when you want to boost your cognitive abilities:

- **Leafy greens.** Leafy greens are important to add to your diet regardless of their cognitive benefits. Leafy greens like kale and broccoli have amazing nutritional value, as they contain vitamin K, fiber, and various other micronutrients. They also have antioxidants that boost your cognitive abilities.

- **Eggs.** Eggs contain a variety of vitamins that are good for your brain health. The most important component found in the egg yolk is choline which helps your neurotransmitters to regulate your emotions and memory. You can also receive B vitamins from eggs, which play a role in synthesizing brain chemicals.

- **Dark chocolate.** Who says that you can't be healthy and enjoy your occasional sweet treats? It's important for you to find healthy treats that provide you with health benefits. Dark chocolate is one of those dessert options you should consider when you want to optimize your brain power. The brain-boosting elements in chocolate include caffeine, antioxidants, and flavonoids. It can enhance your memory and overall boost your mood.

These brain foods will help you to focus, be productive, and enhance your cognitive abilities. If you know that you're going to have a busy mental day, you should ensure that you add these foods to your meals so that you're prepared. Other foods you can include in your diet include oranges, nuts, blueberries, and turmeric, as they can provide you with a brain boost. Oranges improve blood circulation to your brain, nuts boost your memory and learning skills, blueberries reduce your risk of experiencing dementia, and turmeric can stimulate stem cells to produce brain cells.

Supplements to Try

Consuming supplements is one of the best ways to get nutrients into your diet that optimize your cognitive abilities. It's valuable to know which supplements are most effective out there so that you can add them to your diet. These are some of the best supplements you should try and how they can benefit you:

- **Omega-3s.** Omega-3s are fish fats that you find in salmon and sardines, which have a never-ending list of benefits. Unfortunately, most of us can't afford to eat salmon everyday, so eating omega-3s as supplements can provide you with the benefits you need. Your body can't make omega-3s, so it's valuable to consume these supplements to nourish your body with them. These supplements boost the health of your heart, brain, and vision.

- **Magnesium.** If you're struggling with sleeping sufficiently at night and insomnia is something that you suffer from, magnesium can help you to experience better, more restful sleep. Magnesium can also lower your blood pressure and aid blood sugar management. It can reduce your risk of heart disease or migraines, leaving you healthier and more well-rested. This mineral is crucial for the everyday functioning of your body.

- **Multivitamins.** Your body requires all the micronutrients possible, but it can seem extremely overwhelming and even impossible to include them all in your diet. You can't get them all through food, and you don't want to take a handful of supplements every morning. Taking a multivitamin every day can provide you with all of these vitamins you're lacking in your diet. However, multivitamins can be harmful or ineffective if they don't have the right ingredients or dosage for your current eating routine. We will discuss this in more detail further on in the book.

- **Probiotics.** It's highly suggested that you look into consuming probiotics, as they populate your gut with good bacteria. If your gut health is something you've been struggling with, it's time for you to introduce this supplement to your daily diet. If you have an imbalance of good and bad bacteria in your gut, you're at higher risk of experiencing inflammation and certain diseases. This is why it's crucial to populate your gut with good bacteria which causes harmony in your digestive system.

- **Turmeric.** Turmeric is a very accessible supplement that many of us have lying in our cupboards without even realizing the benefits it holds. It's valuable to consume turmeric with fatty foods, as this makes it more likely for them to be absorbed. The anti-inflammatory properties of turmeric can protect your brain against potential diseases, as well as decrease your risk of getting diabetes, kidney disease, or strokes.

Identify the issue you may be facing along your biohacking journey so that you can solve it with the specific supplement that will work best for you. Using supplements like this will solve the issues you may be struggling with along this journey. Try out different types of supplements to experience the best results.

When you're shopping for specific supplements, it's important that you look for the right brands and types that are going to provide you with the most nutritional value. It's important to read labels to ensure your supplements have the appropriate ingredients that will provide you with benefits, instead of exposing you to any harm. We will discuss more details about supplements shortly.

Using Nootropics for Cognitive Advancement

You may know of supplements, as you have used them in the past, but you aren't familiar with nootropics. Nootropics are natural substances that you can use to boost your mental capabilities. They are also known as "smart drugs," as they can improve your focus, better your memory, grasp your attention, and motivate you to be productive and efficient.

They were discovered by a chemist, C. G. Giurgea, who also created piracetam, which is a cognitive boosting smart drug. They've become increasingly popular over the years, as many people swear by them, even big celebrities. For example, Travis Barker is a firm believer in nootropics and their benefits. He uses nootropics to benefit his mood and overall brain functioning. He believes in nootropics so much that he invested in a company that produces nootropics products named "Mindright." Other celebrities like the Jonas Brothers and Bella Hadid swear by nootropics, as they provide them with the cognitive strength and focus they need to be successful in their everyday lives.

We'll discuss some of the best nootropics you can explore for cognitive enhancement shortly.

Nootropics, Supplements, and Techniques for Enhancing Focus, Memory, and Creativity

Hacks and practical techniques aren't the only ways for you to enhance your focus, memory, and creativity, as you can also achieve this with nootropics and supplements. Sometimes we need some help to reach the full potential we desire for ourselves. These "smart drugs" can help you to unlock cognitive capabilities you never knew were possible for you!

The Various Uses for Supplements

When you're following a specific diet, practicing healthy habits, and adjusting your lifestyle to biohacking, you may wonder whether supplements are necessary for your biological advancement. Supplements can be used in various ways to enhance your abilities. Exploring these various solutions can help you to solve some of the physical and mental issues that you've been experiencing. The right supplements can help you in the following aspects of your life:

- **Calming you down.** If stress and anxiety are something you struggle with on a daily basis, consuming the right supplements can help you to achieve a calming effect. You may find that consuming the same calming supplements every day causes you to be a more relaxed individual. These supplements will help you to manage the stress you face in your life, which can boost your health and abilities to fulfill other biohacks in your daily life.

- **More efficient sleep.** We all know how important sufficient sleep is for your well-being. If you try out all of the hacks in the previous chapter, but you still can't get the amount and quality of sleep you desire, supplements may be what you need to achieve deep sleep every night. For example, magnesium will help you to sleep better at night, as we discussed earlier.

- **Complementing specific wellness goals.** Whatever your wellness or fitness goals may be, using supplements can help you to achieve these goals for yourself. For example, you may have a goal that you're able to finish a 5km race. In this case, you can find supplements with vitamin B6, as they help to produce hemoglobin. This allows oxygen to be transported through your blood more efficiently, which ultimately provides you with more energy. There are so many supplements to look into that you're bound to find something that can help you to achieve your wellness goals.

- **Increasing your nutrient intake and improving deficiencies.** Many of us go through life without even realizing that we are deficient in certain vitamins and minerals. Adding supplements to your diet can get rid of these deficiencies that you weren't aware of, which can leave you feeling filled with energy, healthier, and happier.

The benefits of using supplements are never-ending, as they can completely transform your mind and body. You will continuously find something valuable within supplements, as they can be very versatile. Consider some of the ways your diet has been benefiting you and other ways it may be lacking. For these areas that you may be lacking in, it's valuable to find the right supplements that fulfill your needs.

The Value of Nootropics

Though there are various supplements that can help you boost your cognitive and mental capabilities, nootropics have the specific function of boosting your brain health. If you want to go that extra mile when it comes to achieving cognitive capabilities, you will find that using nootropics regularly ensures that you are mentally sharper than you've ever been before. These are some benefits you can expect to receive with nootropics:

- **Better focus.** If being able to focus is something you struggle with, taking nootropics regularly can help you achieve sharper focus and concentration when tackling certain tasks. This allows you to be more productive, as you put all of your energy toward achieving the most optimal outcome for you.

- **Improved memory.** This may not necessarily be something that you struggle with currently, but it will help you to prevent aging in the future. As you grow older, your memory stays sharp and you're at less risk of experiencing dementia and other memory loss related diseases.

- **Increased learning abilities.** Whether you're a student, starting a new job, or you simply want to learn more about life and certain tasks you can accomplish, nootropics can help you to increase your learning abilities. Being more focused and having a better memory helps you to retain the information you learn more effectively.

Nootropics are so valuable, as they provide you with all of these benefits while being safe to use. These "smart drugs" are always backed up by science, which means that they're perfectly curated for your health, without having any harmful side effects. Nootropics have been used for a long time and have had no negative impact on humans, only positive influences.

How to Use Nootropics and Supplements Effectively

When using different supplements, it's important for you to learn how you can use them in the most effective way. If you take them haphazardly without considering the benefits and side effects of each one, you may find that they become entirely ineffective. Knowing how to use supplements and nootropics correctly can help you to experience the most benefits from them.

Supplements That Don't Work Together

There are certain supplements that don't work together, which can make them ineffective when you consume them. You think that you're consuming all of the right supplements that your body needs, but in reality, you're wasting your time and money by pairing the wrong supplements together. It's so important to know which supplements are compatible, and which ones don't work together. These are some popular clashes that you should avoid:

- **Vitamin D, E, and K.** These vitamins are all fat-soluble vitamins that may not be effective taken together in larger doses. Seeing as they are all fat-soluble, only a specific amount of nutrients will be absorbed from these vitamins, as they are all competing to absorb in the presence of fat molecules. You should consume these vitamins separately to avoid ineffective absorption.

- **Iron and calcium.** When you take iron and calcium together, your body is less likely to fully absorb these two vitamins. You should consume iron on an empty stomach to achieve the most effective results.

- **Copper and zinc.** If you have a high level of zinc in your bloodstream, it can result in you having a deficiency of copper. This is why it's crucial to avoid consuming both types of supplements around the same time. However, you should make a habit of including both of these supplements in your diet, as this will provide you with optimal benefits.

- **Certain multivitamins.** Though we said you should explore taking multivitamins so that you can receive all of the nutritional value your body requires, it's important to approach multivitamins with caution. Many of them have vitamin combinations that don't work well together, so it's important to do your research before buying and using just any multivitamin.

When you want to consume any of these supplement combinations, ensure that you're waiting two to three hours before taking the next supplement. With all of these incompatible supplement combinations, it's important for you to be mindful of which supplements you're consuming. You need to ensure that you're pairing the right supplements together for optimal absorption and results.

Supplements to Take Together

As much as there are certain supplements you shouldn't take together, there are also some great supplement combinations that can be more efficient for your supplement journey. Specific vitamins and minerals work really well together, as they help you to absorb nutrients at a faster rate. These are some supplements you can get into the habit of consuming together:

- Vitamin C and zinc
- Calcium and vitamin C
- Vitamin D and omega-3s
- Magnesium and vitamin D
- Magnesium and zinc
- Vitamin C and vitamin B12

When consuming one of the supplements listed above, try to add its compatible component. Doing this will allow you to receive the most benefits from your supplements, as all of the nutrients enter your bloodstream. Don't be afraid of taking multiple supplements at once, just ensure they're compatible and they don't provide you with an overdose of any nutrient.

Supplements to Avoid or Use in Moderation

Though supplements can be really valuable for your mental and physical well-being, there are also some supplements that you should avoid, as they may not be as effective as they appear to be. There is such a thing as too many supplements, as they can be harmful to your internal organs. Knowing which ones you should avoid and which ones to consume in moderation is crucial. These are few you should consider:

- **Vitamin D.** Though vitamin D is crucial for your health and well-being, consuming too much of it can be really unhealthy for your kidneys. Vitamin D supplements are valuable for those who are deficient in this vitamin, but it is suggested for most people to avoid this supplement or consume it in moderation. It's safest to avoid vitamin D supplements, as they can cause abdominal pain, kidney stones, and mood disorders, and even increase your risk of heart attacks. Instead of using supplements, spend an extra 10 to 15 minutes in the sun to receive a healthy dosage of vitamin D.

- **Calcium.** It's always great to include calcium in your supplement diet, as it can strengthen your bones and decrease your risk of suffering from arthritis; however, consuming too much calcium can be bad for you. Some risk factors of too much calcium include hardened arteries, as the excess buildup of calcium can clog your arteries, which gives you a higher risk of suffering from heart diseases. It's important to know what your current calcium levels are in your blood so that you can replenish them with sufficient minerals.

- **St. John's Wort.** This supplement is a plant that you can often use in teas or capsules that provides you with a variety of benefits. It can help you with depression, menopause symptoms, insomnia, wound healing, and kidney and lung issues. However, there is a hidden negative side effect of St. John's Wort that people may not warn you about. When taking this supplement with other medicines, you may find that you have a negative chemical side effect. If you're taking medicine for heart conditions, cancer, or HIV, St. John's Wort can cancel out the important effects of these drugs, which can worsen your preexisting health conditions. For example, if you take St. John's Wort with antidepressants, you may find that you experience blood thinning and an excess of the hormone serotonin, which can cause shivering, diarrhea, and even seizures.

Remember that if any of these specific vitamins and minerals are already in your diet, you shouldn't overkill with supplements. Too much of a good thing can be harmful if you aren't mindful of your consumption. This is why it's so important for you to know the different nutritional value of each food item you consume.

Types of Nootropics

There are various types of nootropics that you can explore. Knowing which type is best for you to try out to experience the results you desire will help you along your biohacking journey. Nootropics can benefit you immensely, as they boost your brain health by protecting your brain, boosting energy levels, balancing the chemicals in your brain, and maintaining and regulating blood flow to the brain. Below are just a few types of nootropics you can explore and the details on how they can boost and enhance your brain health:

- **Vitamins.** As with supplements, nootropics come in specific vitamins that can provide you with the nutrients your mind and body need to function. If you're a beginner to nootropics, exploring your B vitamins can have the greatest benefits on your brain health. Your B-complex vitamins are a great foundation for your nutrients and brain health. Vitamin B6 can help restore memory in older adults, as well as aiding the production of brain chemicals that relieve your stress. Vitamin B9 enhances healthy blood flow to your brain and Vitamin B12 benefits your nervous system by protecting your nerve sheaths. We often don't get enough B vitamins in our diet, so using nootropics will help you to get a more holistic nutritional experience.

- **Herbs.** A more ancient and less modern approach to nootropics is using herbs that have been around for centuries. Certain herbs can have a drastic positive impact on your brain health and capabilities. The modern advancements of these herbs make them more effective and safer for you to add to your diet. Two amazing herbs to try out as a beginner include *Bacopa Monnieri*, which can help you retain knowledge and boost your higher cognitive strengths, and the Lion's Mane Mushroom, which balances your hormones and reduces your risk of cognitive decline as you age. You can purchase fresh lion's mane mushrooms online, but you may find better luck finding the lion's mane mushroom extract in supplement form, as you can find these at your closest drugstore or supermarket. *Bacopa Monnieri* can also be more accessible in supplement form, as you can find it online or at your nearest grocery store. Both of these herbs are also readily available on Amazon.

- **Adaptogens.** Adaptogens are relatively similar to herbs, as they are forms of botanical vegetation that boost your brain's activity. Their main purpose is to aid in the balance of your hormones. A great adaptation to try as a beginner is *Rhodiola Rosea*, as it can calm you down and clear your head. If you find yourself with brain fog or you're overwhelmed by stress, using this adaptogen will help you to feel more at peace and more cognitively aware. As with nootropic herbs, you can find your adaptogens online via stores like Amazon. You can also find a variety of adaptogens readily available at health and wellness stores.

As you explore nootropics, you should try out the various types and discover what benefits you the most. There are various ways your brain can be positively impacted by nootropics. This makes it important for you to identify in which ways your brain power and functioning may be lacking, so you can use the right nootropics to solve this issue. From this, you'll learn what works best for you, so you can integrate it into your diet.

Mindfulness Practices and Meditation for Mental Clarity and Calmness

Being mindful can help you achieve mental clarity and empower you to become the best version of yourself. We can often overlook how powerful our minds truly are, but once you take the time to realize that your mind is in control of your future, you will be able to set realistic goals, stay accountable, and achieve the healthy lifestyle you've always dreamed of for yourself.

Practicing Mindfulness

When you have 101 thoughts racing through your mind, it can be almost impossible to have mental clarity. You struggle to achieve certain tasks, you can't use your cognitive abilities like you thought you could, and you're less productive. Practicing mindfulness can help you achieve the clarity you need to step up your mental game and capabilities.

The stress and chaos of everyday life can make it difficult to remain mindful in the moment. You find yourself so overwhelmed by everyday life that the daily habits you want to develop through biohacking seem impossible. When you're more mindful, you're able to have more clarity and awareness when making the positive changes and transformations you desire. These are some ways you can practice more mindfulness:

- **Focus on one thing at a time.** If you have a lot going on in your life, it can be challenging to be mindful and think with clarity. You're so overwhelmed by a variety of thoughts that you aren't able to make good decisions, practice cognitive skills, and apply critical thinking. Focusing on one task or obstacle at a time can help you to feel more in control mentally.

- **Pay attention to the moment.** Living in the moment can be a lot easier said than done, especially when you find yourself really stressed and overwhelmed. You're constantly thinking about the past or the future, which causes you to neglect your current reality. Paying attention to each moment and living with intention can help you practice the right routines that bring you longevity and health.

- **Mindful habits.** It's time for you to practice your daily habits with more mindfulness. Whether you're practicing positive or negative habits, it's crucial for you to be mindful of the decisions you make and the way you behave. Living life on autopilot can result in resorting to negative habits that aren't fulfilling for you and your biohacking journey.

Being more mindful will help you achieve mental clarity and improved mental performance. You will be surprised to discover how much you're capable of mentally when you remain mindful of your day-to-day lives and capabilities. Being mindful can also help you avoid making any mistakes you may find yourself regretting in the future.

Practicing Meditation

The best way to successfully achieve mental clarity is by being calm. You'll find it challenging to be aware of your thoughts in the moment when you're stressed, overwhelmed, or tense. Practicing meditation regularly can help you achieve a sense of calm that you've been longing for. Being calm and centered within the mind and body will boost your cognitive abilities and improve your daily mental performance. Some other benefits of practicing meditation for biohacking include the following:

- **Increasing your self-awareness.** Meditating regularly can make you a lot more self-aware and mindful. Practicing meditation provides you with special one-on-one time with yourself and your thoughts. You're forced to think about how you feel, certain feelings you may have, and what stressors may be overwhelming you in your life. This helps you to gather a sense of self-awareness that boosts mindfulness and enhances self-improvement.

- **Improving patience and resilience.** For many things in life, having patience is crucial, especially when you're embarking on a journey of transformation. Meditation takes a certain level of patience, as you need to focus, and you won't receive results overnight. This learned skill of patience will help you to approach this journey with a healthy mindset, as you aren't rushing the process.

- **Becoming less dependent on addictions.** When you meditate frequently, you may find that it's an effective tool that helps you to let go of addictions. Whenever you find yourself reverting back to an addiction that harms you, you can use meditation as a tool to be more mindful and resilient in that moment. Once you're done with meditation, you may think twice about practicing addictive habits. Of course, overcoming addiction is not easy, so seek professional help. However, practicing meditation frequently will help you to manage your addictions and cravings.

These are only a few benefits you can receive from meditating regularly, as there are many more ways meditation will transform your life when you give it a fair trial. We will explore meditation in more depth throughout the next chapter. You'll discover different types of meditation and specific meditation techniques that can provide you with the best outcomes.

Enhancing Cognitive Behavior with Technology

Supplements and nootropics aren't the only ways you can advance your cognitive abilities, as using cutting-edge technologies can allow you to reach your full potential. Your mind is capable of so much more when you use biohacking innovation and technology to advance yourself!

Neurofeedback

Neurofeedback is a form of therapy that allows you to understand how your brain responds to stressors, by studying your brain waves. It is used to help you manage how you handle stress in your day-to-day life. It connects your mind and body, allowing you to stay calm, instead of triggering your fight-or-flight response. However, neurofeedback isn't just used to manage your anxiety, it can also help to manage PTSD, ADHD, autism, depression, and insomnia.

Going to the source of your brain allows you to transform the way your receptors respond to certain situations. Neurofeedback is performed by placing sensors on your scalp that monitor and process your brain waves. A medical professional will then use this data to create a specific program that targets your negative stress responses. They alter your brain waves to improve your brain functionality and patterns so that you can experience more heightened cognitive capabilities like concentration, brainstorming, problem-solving, and organization.

Brain Simulation

One of the most scientifically advanced innovations to date is brain simulation, as it is the practice of researchers and scientists making computer models of the complex brain. Though it's complicated, it's a necessary form of technology that helps us know more about how the brain works.

With this knowledge, we can experience a future of better health and technological advancements as biohackers. Brain simulations will provide us with specialized knowledge and data that allow us to develop specific treatments and strategies to tackle disorders, health issues, and neurodegenerative diseases.

Cognitive Training Apps

One of the most convenient ways to sharpen your cognitive skills is by making use of cognitive training apps. We spend most of our days on our phones, so why not spend that time practicing some enriching exercises that can boost your cognitive abilities? Some great cognitive training apps you can explore include the following:

- **Elevate.** This app provides you with over 30 games that can test your intelligence and mental capacity. You challenge various cognitive skills such as memory, comprehension, concentration, and math.

- **Lumosity.** Lumosity also tests various skills such as mental speed, memory, attention span, and problem-solving. It also tracks your data and shows you your improvement over time.

- **Cognito.** If you're looking for more game-like activities that stimulate your brain, while entertaining you,

Cognito is the app for you. It uses fun games to measure your logic, memory, and focus.

As with most cognitive training apps, these apps allow you to download and play for free, but if you want to unlock more features, you'll need to pay for a premium subscription. Due to the variety of apps you can find online, you can use different cognitive training apps each day to achieve the best results. Constantly challenging your mind with different exercises will keep you mentally sharp, and focused, and will boost your memory.

Chapter 5:

Managing Stress and Optimizing Emotional and Mental Well-Being

Stress doesn't have to control your life any longer, as you are the master of your mind and your destiny. When you take the proper measures to manage your stress, you will discover how much it optimizes your emotional and mental well-being. Looking after your mental health will help you to adopt a mindset that encourages you to put your health and longevity first.

Through this chapter, you will understand the stress response more, as you discover lifestyle modifications that can enhance your emotional and mental well-being. Working toward long-term mental health and happiness will allow you to enjoy a lifestyle that is rewarding, instead of overwhelming and stressful.

The Relationship Between Stress and Biohacking

The ultimate objective of biohacking is to nurture and nourish your body in a way that you thrive and become the best version of yourself both physically and mentally. You want to live a long, happy, and fulfilling life where you're able to accomplish as many tasks and activities as possible, without having stress distracting you from your journey.

The Impact of Stress on the Mind

Continuous stress can take a huge toll on your mental well-being, as it is a strenuous mindset that is constantly worrying you. This can be especially taxing when you're experiencing a large transformation in your life. These are just a few ways stress can be strenuous for your mind:

- **Increases your risk of mental health disorders.** Stressing regularly can dramatically increase your risk of getting mental health disorders such as anxiety and depression. Experiencing mental health issues decreases your quality of life drastically. If you find yourself struggling with anxiety or depression, it's important to seek professional help, as your mental health issues should not be taken lightly. Being able to manage your stress effectively will decrease your risk of developing these disorders.

- **Unhealthy cognitive aging.** If you are currently stressed every day, you may not discover any cognitive repercussions at the moment, but as you age, you may find yourself struggling cognitively. Your memory deteriorates, you have less mental sharpness, and you aren't able to accomplish as many tasks as you wish you could.

- **Feeling mentally exhausted.** Constantly stressing about something in your life is not only strenuous to your mind, but it can also be a really unpleasant experience emotionally. You're so tired of always worrying about something, and the constant stress leaves you at the edge of your seat. As much as you try to be positive and manage your stress, your worries become the focal point of your mental state.

Experiencing intense stress can make it seem impossible to become the best version of yourself. You are so entirely overwhelmed by your thoughts that you can't think positively about yourself and your future. This prevents you from taking the necessary steps you need to grow.

The Impact of Stress on The Body

Stress doesn't only take a toll on you mentally, but it can also drastically impact you physically. This impact on your body makes it challenging for you to achieve everything you desire through biohacking. These are just a few ways stress may be negatively impacting your body:

- **Gut health issues.** Have you ever been really overwhelmed by your stress and anxiety and your stomach starts to feel really funny? It feels as though you need to rush to the toilet, you have lots of pent-up gas, or your stomach just feels strange. Stressing regularly can take a toll on your gut health as it can cause inflammation in your gut.

- **Neglecting self-care.** When you find yourself really preoccupied with stress and anxiety, you may neglect self-care. Looking after your body is so important, especially when you want it to thrive in health and strength. When you're overwhelmed by stress, doing small self-care tasks can feel huge.

- **Tense and sore muscles.** You've had a stressful week at work and all you can wish for is a nice long massage. Your muscles have been tense non-stop, even when you go to sleep. This can be quite painful after some time, as you develop knots and strains from being so tense with stress.

You won't be able to train and hack your body to its best biological ability, as the stress of life takes a toll on you. Doing simple tasks can feel impossible and you find yourself getting sick and injured too often for you to make the proper progress that you desire. It's also important to realize that consistent stress for a large portion of your life can actually result in a lower life expectancy, as it can put you more at risk of health issues and diseases. To live a life of health and longevity, you need to ensure that your stress doesn't take over your life anymore.

Effective Stress Management Techniques

Knowing how to manage your stress will be a game-changer for you when you're taking on the biohacking world. Stress can often take over our entire being, so it's important to remember that you are in control! Practicing these stress management techniques can help you conquer your anxiety once and for all!

Embrace Nature

You've been spending most of your time in the office working diligently, at home getting housework done, and if you get some physical activity done, you're doing it in a gym. Spending most of your time inside an enclosed environment can actually increase your risk of suffering from anxiety.

We all need to spend some time outdoors embracing nature, as it can help us to become grounded and present in the moment. If you find yourself feeling really overwhelmed, you may find it effective to embrace nature for a bit. These are some simple ways you can embrace nature and become stress-free:

- **Go for walks.** If you're feeling really stressed and overwhelmed, these don't have to be intense walks, as they can be slow strolls, as long as you're surrounded by some sense of nature. Going for walks in nature can kill two birds with one stone, as you embrace nature, while getting some exercise done. Making this a daily routine that you use to either start or end your day will help you feel a lot less stressed.

- **Enjoy nature with loved ones.** Nature can be even more enjoyable to embrace when you're surrounded by loved ones. Forget about eating at restaurants, going to the mall, or staying home and watching Netflix all day. Being surrounded by loved ones in nature can help you to build a deeper connection with them. Go to the park or the beach and have a picnic with friends or family. Go on hikes together, or practice other activities that allow you to embrace the rawness of nature.

- **Centering yourself in nature.** If you've been longing to develop a deeper connection with nature, as you want to be one with nature, meditating in a natural and scenic location can help you to feel calmer than ever before. It's just you and nature as you connect with your surroundings and develop a deeper sense of belonging. You can practice mindfulness, take in your scenic surroundings, or meditate in a natural setting to really feel more connected with nature.

- **Bathe in the sun.** One of the main reasons why you should be embracing the outdoors is so that you can get a dosage of vitamin D. As we discussed previously, vitamin D is so crucial for your overall health and well-being. Sitting in the sun for 10 to 15 minutes can do wonders for your mood. You'll find yourself feeling more positive and stress-free afterward. Doing this on a daily basis will have a huge positive impact on your health, as you get sufficient vitamin D without having to rely on supplements.

These are simply a few ideas that can inspire you to explore and embrace nature in your own way. You could try out these activities or experience nature in its natural form by sitting in a scenic location and taking in your surroundings. Just a few minutes outdoors will do wonders for your mental well-being. When you really start to appreciate and love nature, you will find that you live a higher quality life.

Meditation

As we briefly discussed previously, meditation is a crucial exercise you should practice to relieve yourself of stress and anxiety. There are various ways to practice and benefit from meditation. It's just about finding the best techniques for you that will biohack your mind and body. Exploring these different types of meditation can help you to find something that works best for you:

- **Body scan meditation.** To meditate and bring more awareness to your mind and body, you should practice this body scan meditation technique. Start by lying down with your back on the floor and closing your eyes. Tense your whole body and release it. Now it's time to focus on each part of your body, as you use the squeeze and release method. Starting at your feet, make the muscles in your feet tense, squeeze your toes, and roll your ankles. After doing this for a few seconds, you can then release your feet muscles and completely relax them. From this, you move on to your calves and proceed to practice the same method on each part of your body, until your entire body feels really relaxed. Ensure that you also practice this technique on your face, as you make your face tense and then completely relax. This form of meditation helps you to let go of any tension you may be feeling in your body while bringing awareness to yourself and distracting your mind from your worries.

- **Mindfulness meditation.** If you find that your mind has been distracted lately and you can't seem to focus on what's important, you should practice mindfulness meditation. This form of meditation influences you to take a look into your mind and channel your thoughts to something more mindful and constructive. This should be a judge-free zone where you bring your awareness to your thoughts and find ways to transform them into more positive and enriching thoughts. Take some time to yourself in a quiet location, close your eyes, and think about everything that may be stressing and overwhelming you. Ensure that you're mindful of each thought and give yourself the opportunity to understand each thought process. As you think these thoughts, consider how they make you feel, how they impact your body, and determine whether you're mindful of your breath or not.

- **Movement meditation.** If you try your best to stay still and focused as you meditate, but you aren't getting anywhere because of your lack of focus, practicing movement meditation may be just what you need. Going for a walk while meditating can help you to achieve a sense of zen and focus that you may not have achieved at home with your distracting thoughts. You can even practice meditation as you exercise. A common form of exercise people practice for meditative purposes is yoga, as it is a physical activity that helps you to achieve a sense of zen and meditative state. Wherever you're practicing movement meditation, be sure to maintain mindfulness of your breath, as this will allow you to enter a meditative and focused state.

Meditating successfully can be a lot easier said than done, as you find yourself being easily distracted or struggling to discover your inner zen. Ensuring that you're in a good environment, your mind is focused, and you eliminate any external distractions will ensure that you have the best meditation experience possible!

Aromatherapy

Aromatherapy is the practice of using essential oils to create a therapeutic effect. Our senses can be very powerful, especially the sense of smell. We can often overlook our sense of smell, but it can be quite relaxing. This is what you'll experience and explore with aromatherapy. These are some ways you can use aromatherapy:

- **Diffuser.** A diffuser is a common method used generally to experience aromatherapy. Use a device that breaks essential oils into smaller particles, so they surround you in the air. You can leave the diffuser on with different essential oils for different occasions and benefits.

- **Steam.** To have a more concentrated version of your essential oils in the air, you should pursue the steaming method. You start off by boiling a pot of water and removing it from the heat, adding your essential oils. You should only be adding three to five drops of essential oils. You can then place your head over it, with a towel draped over your head to trap in all of the heat. Ensure that the steam is not so hot that it could hurt you.

- **Aroma stick.** If you want to have an aromatherapy option that is portable, the aroma stick is for you. It's a plastic stick with a wick at the end which contains your essential oils. You leave it covered when not using it, but when you're in need of aromatherapy, you can uncover it and take a sniff, experiencing all of its relieving powers.

If you're doing aromatherapy on your own, you should be mindful when shopping for essential oils. Buying just any essential oils can result in you having a less effective and immersive experience. Some helpful ways for you to purchase the right essential oils is by doing the following:

- **Read the label.** To ensure that the essential oils you're buying are legitimate, you must read the labels and see if they have all of the necessary information. Labels tell you all you need to know about essential oils. Look out for the plants used in the essential oil, their growth method, and the various contents of the oil. Most importantly, check if they are organic, as this means they are more high-quality.

- **Avoid fragranced oils.** Essential oils with fragrances are often not as effective as they may appear. Fragranced essential oils often have added chemicals that can be harmful. You want to buy oils that are 100% pure, as these will be most effective for you.

- **Compare products.** Don't buy the first essential oils that you see in the store. You want to search for quality and affordability. The more you look around and compare products, the more likely you are to find the most suitable essential oils that you can trust for years to come.

Once you've discovered the right essential oils for you, it's time for you to buy the right ones that will provide you with the most calming effect. You might have to shop around and discover what works best for you, but once you know which types and brands of essential oils work best for you, you will experience optimal results from aromatherapy.

Lastly, to ensure that you are using the right combinations to receive a calming effect from essential oils, consider some of these winning blends. Using these effective combinations will ensure that you have the best results from aromatherapy:

- **Lavender, chamomile, and ylang ylang.** Making a blend including five drops of lavender, three drops of chamomile, and one drop of ylang ylang can leave you with a scent that balances your moods and helps you deal with anxiety and stress.

- **Bergamot, sandalwood, and clary sage.** A blend including five drops of sandalwood, three drops of clary sage, and one drop of bergamot can help you to feel more grounded and connected with yourself as you meditate or practice yoga.

- **Peppermint, rosemary, and lavender.** Adding five drops of lavender, three drops of rosemary, and two drops of peppermint to your diffuser can provide you with an energizing aroma that can lift you up when you're feeling a bit down or overwhelmed.

- **Juniper berry, rosemary, and grapefruit.** A blend containing five drops of grapefruit, three drops of juniper berry, and two drops of rosemary can help you battle the negative emotions you may be experiencing with your anxiety.

There are a variety of blends you can use for different purposes and levels of effectiveness. If you're looking for that calming effect, these should be your go-to blends. Try out as many of these combinations as you can, to determine what works best for you!

Breathwork

One of the most effective ways for you to relieve yourself of stress is by focusing your attention on controlling your breath. When you're feeling really stressed, you may find that your breath is out of control, you struggle to breathe, and your breaths are very short as you hyperventilate.

Taking a step back and being able to control your breath can help you to calm down drastically. We've discussed how to use breathwork via meditation, but there are some other effective ways for you to use breathwork to your advantage. When you find yourself really stressed and overwhelmed in the moment, you can use breathwork exercises to calm you down. Here are some simple breathwork exercises you can explore for the most calming results:

- **Breath focus.** When you're feeling really anxious and overwhelmed, the best thing for you to do is bring your focus back to your breath entirely. Forget about the stressors around you that may be causing you to hyperventilate, and only have your mind set on how you're inhaling and exhaling oxygen. Start by breathing normally to identify how each inhale and exhale makes you feel. You can then take deeper breaths by inhaling to the count of three, holding for a beat, and then exhaling to the count of three. As you practice this deep breathing, you should repeat a word that brings you a sense of comfort and peace, for example, safe or calm.

- **Abdominal breathing.** You may be used to practicing deep breathing by using your chest, but to get a deeper, more effective breathing experience, you should try abdominal breathing, also known as belly breathing. As you inhale, ensure that you're filling your belly with air. Place your hands on your abdomen to feel it expand. Hold your breath for a beat and then exhale fully. Feel your abdomen deflate. Repeat this a couple of times until you start to feel a sense of calm and ensure that you are focusing on breathing with your abdomen for the entirety of the breathing exercise.

- **Lion's breath.** To embrace a breathing exercise that makes you feel more self-confident and empowered, the lion's breath is the most optimal form of breathwork for you. You're able to let go of anxiety holding you back; as you breathe you release all of your insecurities and frustrations with each exhale. Sit cross-legged, placing your hands on your knees. Sit up straight and inhale deeply through your nose. As you exhale, let out a "ha" with your mouth wide open and your tongue stretched as far out as possible. Repeat this breathing style several times.

When practicing any of these breathing exercises, it's important for you to be mindful and aware of your breath and how it makes you feel. The breath is so powerful—feel it filling your body, giving you life, and releasing the stress that is stored in your mind and body. Try out all of these breathing exercises and discover which one works best for you whenever you find yourself in a stressful situation.

Use a Journal

We've discussed how you can use a food journal to benefit you along your biohacking journey, but journals can be used for a variety of purposes. You can use a journal for personal reasons to clear your head and help you manage your stress more effectively. Sometimes all we need to do is express our thoughts and worries so that we can move on with a sense of peace and calm. Here are some valuable ways to use a journal to benefit you along your journey:

- **Reflecting on your day.** Being able to reflect on your day-to-day life through your journal can tell you a lot about your thoughts and how you feel. As you reflect on your day through your journal, you can explore how you used biohacking during your day. Record the various emotions, thoughts, and behaviors you've experienced throughout the day.

- **Writing down stressors and frustrations.** When you experience something really stressful and overwhelming, turning to your journal can help you unleash all of your stress and anxiety. Instead of letting your thoughts get overwhelmed by stress, consider writing down your frustrations and expressing them in this way. Remember that it's your journal, so you can write down anything you want about your day, feelings, or frustrations.

- **Writing down positive affirmations.** To release your stress, you also need to replace your mind and thoughts with positive thinking. Writing down positive affirmations on a daily basis can help you feel better about yourself. Your journal shouldn't just be about negative feelings, as you want to integrate some positivity that brightens your mood and makes you feel motivated.

- **Seeing your progress.** Getting a journal and writing in it frequently can help you discover how much progress you're making along your journey. Seeing how far you've come and the progress you're making will make you feel more motivated to be consistent and continuously push yourself as a biohacker. You can record the negative days you may experience that make you feel like giving up, so you can look back at them and feel proud for continuously pushing yourself.

Though journaling may seem like something so simple, it is really effective. It can help you feel as though you're in more control of your life throughout the most stressful and overwhelming circumstances. Getting your thoughts out on paper can be therapeutic, which allows you to tackle each task with more strength and resilience.

Chapter 6:

Biohacking for Longevity and Healthy Aging

The greatest goal for most of us is to live a long and healthy life. You can create that future for yourself through discipline and motivation. Envisioning a long and healthy future can keep you going on your biohacking journey, as you establish what you need to do to make this your reality. You can live a long, healthy, and happy life if you really make the effort to adjust your habits.

Aging doesn't have to be something that you dread and fear. You can approach old age knowing that you're going to be as healthy and active as you can possibly be. When you age gracefully, you're able to truly enjoy your senior years, by having the ability to do all the tasks you've always wanted to. You can be independent, without needing anyone to take care of you every day.

Exploring the Relationship Between Biohacking and Longevity

The objective of biohacking is to live a long and fulfilling lifestyle. Your goal should be to unlock your biological potential through effective hacks and techniques. When you become the best version of yourself physically and mentally, you'll be able to live a long and fulfilling life of independence and health.

Living a Life of Longevity

When you practice biohacks regularly and create a healthy biohacking routine, you're bound to live a longer, more enriching life. These healthy habits are ultimately what allows you to live the long life that you desire, as you're less likely to suffer from diseases, you're able to stay physically fit at an old age, and you don't experience extreme fatigue and even feelings of dread.

Health, especially in your old age, is not something you pay for. Many people approach this stage of their lives wishing they were healthier and more capable of living a good quality of life, but it can often be too late.

Aging Gracefully

Not only do you experience a long and enriching life, but you also find that the aging process is a lot more graceful. No matter what age you are, you get to live life to the fullest, without having your age hold you back in life. These are some reasons why aging is so enjoyable for biohackers:

- **Having independence.** One of the worst parts of aging is lacking the independence to live life how you normally would when you were younger. Independence is something many of us can take for granted when we're younger, but when we have to rely on others during old age, we become aware of how valuable it truly is. Being independent in your old age will allow you to live life to the fullest no matter what, which makes life so much more enjoyable.

- **Lower risk of suffering from diseases and conditions.** Old age can be a painful stage of life for many, as they experience diseases and medical conditions that can drastically decrease their quality of life. You don't have to wake up with aches or pains or suffer discomfort as a side effect of illnesses or conditions. This will make old age more enjoyable for you, as you don't have to struggle with your health.

- **Being mentally sharp.** When you look after your mind and body now, you'll approach old age with a sharp and aware mind. Many individuals who approach old age find themselves struggling, as they experience memory loss, their cognitive abilities decrease, and they aren't as mentally sharp as they once used to be. This can make it challenging for you to get through day-to-day life on your own, as you're constantly forgetting or finding yourself incapable of critical thinking.

Many of us dread aging, as we want to enjoy youth for as long as possible, but aging shouldn't be something you fear, especially when you're practicing biohacks that can allow you to age gracefully. You can still make the most of your day-to-day life, remain physically active, find pleasure in the outdoors, and move around independently. All you need to do is start transforming your lifestyle now with biohacking!

Anti-Aging Approaches, Cellular Optimization, and Methods for Promoting Healthy Aging

The world of biohacking can expose you to some of the most modern and innovative approaches to anti-aging. You may worry a lot about aging, or it may not even be a thought of yours, as you're still young. Regardless of your thoughts and opinions, pursuing anti-aging now will benefit you in the long run. Practicing these methods regularly will provide you with long-term results that allow you to be the best version of yourself, even when you're 80.

Lifestyle Factors That Contribute to a Long Life

Transforming your lifestyle for the better is what can help you achieve the long and fulfilling life that you desire for yourself. We've discussed many of them already throughout the book such as avoiding smoking, and alcohol, sleeping sufficiently, and eating a healthy diet. However, there are some other great lifestyle factors that you must consider if you want to live a long and fulfilling life. These are a few of them:

Exercising Regularly

We've discussed how important exercise is for you if you want to achieve your physical and biological goals. Exercising frequently will also help you to live a long and healthy life. You need to train your body on a daily basis to get to a physical fitness level that promotes a long and healthy life. It can be challenging to commit yourself to exercise every day, as you're going to have days where you feel lazy and disinterested in physical exercise. Some effective ways to ensure that you're exercising regularly include the following:

- **Doing an exercise that makes you happy.** If you are doing a certain sport or exercise that you don't enjoy, you're probably not going to commit your time to it by practicing it frequently. Try out different forms of exercise to discover what brings you the most joy. You can pursue sports where you play with others, go to the gym, go for runs, or try out specific athletic sports like CrossFit.

- **Finding people to exercise with.** Sometimes exercising alone can be really dull and boring. Having close friends and family to exercise with will motivate you to get going and have fun. Each experience with physical activity will be more enjoyable, which motivates you to keep going.

- **Set physical goals.** When you have a grand physical goal that you'd like to reach in your life, you will find yourself feeling more motivated. You want to accomplish your goals, so you're going to work hard and be consistent. For example, you may set a physical goal that you want to be able to do 30 pull-ups, so to achieve this, you need to continuously train your upper body. Setting goals will make you more likely to stay committed and accountable to the fitness aspect of your life.

Once you find a specific routine and way of exercising that is most suitable for you, you will be more likely to stick to this as a lifestyle. You'll look forward to exercising every day, as it provides you with a sense of peace and joy.

Play Brain Games

When your goal is to live a long, productive, and healthy life, you need to keep your mind enriched and healthy through specific games and tools. Challenging brain games can keep you mentally sharp and focused, as you have to use different parts of your brain to solve these complex problems. These are some effective brain games you can explore to boost your brain health and longevity:

- **Sudoku and crossword.** Some common brain game activities that everyone thinks of automatically are sudoku and crosswords. Though they may seem simple and old-fashioned, sudoku and crosswords can get those brain muscles warmed up and activated, so it's a great place for you to start. If you enjoy numbers, sudoku is for you, but if you're more of a words person, explore some fun crosswords.

- **Problem-solving questions.** A great way to challenge your mind and keep it occupied is by practicing some problem-solving skills that challenge you. Finding some problems online or via apps can get your brain juices flowing, as you explore some of the most difficult problems. Practicing problem-solving can help you to improve your cognitive skills in various aspects of your life. You may even find it easier to solve problems in your professional or personal life.

- **Download brain games apps.** Fortunately, there are hundreds and thousands of different and unique brain games apps available for you to download. It's time for you to take advantage of technology and download some apps that will challenge your mind. You can explore different types of brain games, with a variety of levels of difficulty, depending on how much you want to challenge yourself. Switching between a variety of these games keeps you interested and engaged.

Constant practice will strengthen those brain muscles! So, the more you practice these brain games, the more it will benefit you in the future cognitively. Again, it's important to note that you can explore brain games and technology. Don't limit yourself to physical brain game exercises like sudoku books, as there's a world of problem-solving digitally for you to uncover!

Hormone Replacement Therapy

Hormone replacement therapy (HRT) is used to manage imbalanced hormones. This practice is most often used to balance the hormones of women going through menopause, which in return can reduce the symptoms they experience. If you are experiencing this hormonal imbalance in your life, you may find that it makes you more stressed, negative, and irritable, and your body doesn't function to its optimal capabilities.

Hormone replacement therapy is a great solution for women struggling with hormonal imbalance, as a woman's menstrual cycle can contribute to a vast fluctuation of the hormones estrogen and progesterone. Some benefits of participating in hormone replacement therapy include reducing negative symptoms of menopause and hormonal imbalances, lowered risk of suffering from osteoporosis, relieved joint pain, and a reduced risk of getting diabetes. There is even a lower death rate of women in their fifties who take HRT!

However, there are also risk factors that come with HRT such as being at higher risk of experiencing potential blood clots, gallbladder issues, strokes, and endometrial cancer. If you're considering trying out hormone therapy, it is best for you to seek professional advice and treatment. A doctor can provide you with the optimal form of HRT through diagnosis.

Exploring Cutting Edge Technology

If you take advantage of technological inventions, devices, and strategies, you will find that your quality of life drastically improves. You give yourself more power to enjoy life to the fullest while exploring advancements that can allow you to live a longer and healthier life. These are some forms of cutting-edge technology you should explore:

- **Senescence reversal.** Senescence is damaged cells that contribute to aging, aesthetics, and even weakened immunity. Biohackers believe in rejuvenating cells to ensure longevity, health, and anti-aging, which is disrupted by senescent cells. It is thought that reversed senescence can help you to live longer and reduce your aging symptoms. Senescence reversal can be achieved through consuming senolytic drugs which you can purchase online. Senolytic drugs contain a special protein that promotes anti-aging. Another way to achieve senescence reversal can be through stem cell therapy.

- **Stem cell therapy.** Stem cells are original and raw cells in your body that can fulfill a variety of functions. Stem cell therapy is the practice of using stem cells to rejuvenate and heal your body, as these cells can regenerate. It's a natural and effective way to repair your body and reach your physical performance and health goals. If you are interested in exploring stem cell therapy, you should visit a professional like Novastem, as they use the latest stem cell therapy technology to set up a framework that allows you to become the healthiest version of yourself.

- **Gene editing.** Gene editing is a scientific practice that alters your DNA. There are gene editing equipment and tools that biohackers use to manipulate and alter their genes. This biohack can be successful when practiced by a professional, but when it comes to DIY gene editing, you need to be extra cautious, and research-focused. Not every biohacker has had a successful experience with gene editing. Josiah Zayner, a well-known biohacker who is a CEO of a biotech company, has always pushed the limits with biohacking but found himself going too far. At a live event, he injected himself with a CRISPR kit and received a ton of backlash for dangerously promoting a kit that wasn't approved by the FDA yet. He performed this act, thinking it would result in muscle growth, but was shortly disappointed.

Making use of these innovations can allow you to live a longer, more fulfilling life. There are so many ways you can integrate technology into your life through biohacking, which we will discuss in greater detail in Chapter 8.

Chapter 7:

Personalizing Your Biohacking Routine

You now know of various biohacking strategies and techniques that may be good for you and your progress, but how do they apply to your life and your body? It's important to remember that this entire biohacking journey is for you, which means you need to personalize it to get the most out of it! You deserve that extra thought and consideration to make a routine that suits your wants and needs. It's time to put yourself first by customizing biohacking to your lifestyle.

Customizing Your Biohacking Routine

As we've discussed throughout the book, it's crucial for you to personalize your biohacking routine so that it suits your body and its needs. Merely following general biohacking techniques and strategies won't help you achieve the true results you desire. To make your routine more personal to you and your needs, consider the following tips:

Identify Your Personal Goals

The first step to personalizing your biohacking routine is identifying the goals you want for yourself and your future. Whether you're fully aware of it or not, there's a specific reason why you're reading this book. You want to advance yourself biologically in a specific way, but you're unsure how to achieve this. It's crucial for you to identify and be aware of these goals before getting started, as this is what you need to keep in mind for the duration of your biohacking journey.

When you know what your personal and holistic goals are along this journey, you'll be able to take the right measures to make them a reality. If you don't have any specific goals in mind currently, you can answer these questions to discover what you want from this journey:

- **What physical goals do you have?** We all have specific goals that we want to meet in our lives in terms of physicality, whether we're aware of it or not. Take a second to consider some of the physical goals you've desired for yourself, whether it's appearance-wise or ability-wise. It may be something specific like being able to run a marathon, or it could be something general like wanting to better your health and fitness. You can also set health goals for yourself if you're struggling with illnesses or negative recurring symptoms.

- **What type of lifestyle do you want for yourself?** The lifestyle you desire has a big impact on the types of biohacking you should pursue. Think about your dream lifestyle that you've always wanted to live, but you've never had the opportunity. What you want your day-to-day life to look like can tell you a lot about the direction you should go with biohacking. Advancing yourself biologically can help you gain the mental sharpness and physical strength that allows you to live the lifestyle you long for.

- **What are some aspects of your current life you'd like to improve?** Take a look at the day-to-day life you're currently living. Identifying what you like and dislike about your current routine and daily outcomes can help you determine where you should seek improvement. Be completely honest with yourself about what you dislike and the weaknesses that are setting you back in your life. For example, you may really dislike procrastinating at work, as it prevents you from excelling. In this case, biohacking can help you to advance your concentration and productivity levels.

- **What do you want your future to look like?** When you dream of a prosperous and successful future, what are some of the details and thoughts you have toward this future? When you think about what you want, you may be too realistic or pessimistic, which causes you to doubt or downplay what you truly want your future to look like. Consider the dream future you want for yourself and how biohacking can get you there. For example, you may want to approach old age fitter than ever, so you can travel the world. Biohacking can help you to explore longevity through healthy eating and effective practices.

Throughout your biohacking journey, it's crucial for you to prioritize your overall health, but you should mainly focus on accomplishing the goals you set for yourself. When you use biohacking to achieve your wildest dreams and goals, you'll feel more fulfilled and satisfied along this journey. Biohacking isn't easy, but if it's helping you to achieve your wildest dreams, you'll be more likely to stick to it.

Experiment with Biohacking and Your Body

In order to create a personalized biohacking routine that works for you, you need to be willing to experiment with your body, by trying various biohacks. You may avoid certain biohacks, as you think that they won't be effective for you, but you never know how some techniques will work until you give them a fair try. These are some more effective ways to experiment with your body and biohacking:

- **Adapt biohacks.** Remember that with all of these biohacks you've read and some new ones you may learn about, you can create your own rules and regulations and adapt them to your liking. Biohacks may not work specifically for you, as your body doesn't effectively function with these techniques and strategies. This is why it's valuable to adapt and experiment with biohacks so that they're most suitable for you.

- **Thinking outside of the box.** As we've discussed, it's important to try out a variety of new biohacks to see what works best for you. Instead of just trying what other biohackers do, it's valuable to think outside of the box, while still considering the concept of biohacking. For example, you could create a specialized protein-focused diet that is all vegan. Experimenting can expose you to some life-changing results. Some of the most successful biohackers are those who think outside of the box and come up with biohacks that set them apart biologically.

Along this journey, it's important for you to really push yourself out of your comfort zone. You never know what your body is truly capable of if you don't experiment with biohacking. The more you embrace these changes, the more you'll learn about your body and what it needs.

Trial and Error

As you explore with your body while experimenting with various biohacks, you should embrace the trial-and-error method. The goal is to try out a variety of biohacks and practices, seeing which ones work for you. You can discover what doesn't work for you and eliminate it from your biohacking lifestyle. Stick to using biohacks that show you promising results. As you explore trial and error with biohacking, you should consider the following tips:

- **Record all progress.** In order to determine whether a biohack is successfully working for you or not, you need to be able to record all of the progress you make. This is where a journal comes into play, as you can write down all of the biohacks you explore, how you responded to them, and the continuous progress or lack thereof that you receive from them. You need to refer back to this book for each biohack so that you can determine what's working for you or what's not. It's important to record every detail you experience when making modifications to your diet and lifestyle so that you have an accurate perception of how the biohacks are working for you.

- **Give each biohack a fair trial.** When pursuing and practicing different biohacks, it's crucial for you to give each biohack a fair and equal chance. You may find a certain biohack more challenging than the others, which makes you feel like giving up and moving on to something else. It's important for you to give each biohack a proper try, even if it's not providing you with immediate results. Practice it over a decent period of time to receive a more accurate outcome.

- **Revisit biohacks.** Just because a biohack hasn't worked for you in the past, doesn't mean it will always be ineffective. Our bodies evolve and change, especially when we introduce ourselves to a new lifestyle. If you find that you haven't tried a specific biohack in a while, you can retry it to see how it may benefit you now. You may find that being a more experienced biohacker makes certain biohacks easier to use and more effective for you.

Once you successfully practice trial and error, you will identify the best biohacking practices for you, and avoid biohacks that simply don't work for your body. Doing this will allow you to find the specific biohacks that work for you, which will ultimately allow you to put together a routine most suitable for you.

Download Your Planner

To help you stay on track and focused along your biohacking journey, you will find a free downloadable planner attached to this book. This planner can not only allow you to stay accountable and goal-driven, but it can also help you to find ways to personalize your biohacking journey perfectly for you! You'll be able to download it via a link at the end of this book.

Chapter 8:

Advanced Biohacking Technologies and Trends

It's time to explore some of the most advanced biohacking technologies out there. Biohacking is growing and evolving each day, so keeping up to date with cutting-edge technology can improve your success rate with this methodology. As technology and science develop, new innovations are created that can make our lives more convenient and healthier. Exploring these fascinating and groundbreaking trends will inspire you to embrace biohacking and all of the opportunities it has for you!

Exploring Cutting-Edge Biohacking Technologies, Gadgets, Practices, and Devices.

Gadgets and devices can be used to enhance any and every aspect of your life. We're fortunate to live in an era where so much technology is available to us, so it's time for you to embrace the opportunity to take advantage of it throughout your biohacking journey.

Biohacking Blood Tests

Doing blood tests can help you to determine a lot about your health and any issues or deficiencies you may have. It can give you a more accurate result on your body and what you may require to achieve your full biological potential. Your blood can tell you everything about your health, which can be a massive help for your biohacking implementation. Here are some other ways doing a blood test can help you receive the best results along your biohacking journey:

- **Discovering what vitamins you need.** When you do a blood test, you can identify the vitamins and minerals your body is lacking, and what nutrients you need to solve any of the issues you may be facing. For example, if you're feeling really drained and you're struggling to sleep at night, it may be a sign that you need magnesium in your diet. A blood test can confirm or deny this theory. From the data you discover you can decide how to integrate these nutrients into your diet, either through food or supplements.

- **Learning about health issues.** Doing a blood test can actually uncover potential health issues you may have that have been causing a decline in your well-being. You'll also feel more validated when taking a blood test, as you understand why you always feel so tired or sick. You realize you're not crazy, as your body is just asking for specific nutrients and care. You can work toward solving these health issues and boost your overall well-being with biohacking.

- **Helping your trial-and-error journey.** If you want to discover how biohacks are working for your body, doing a blood test can give you accurate results. You can learn whether your new eating habits are working for you or not, by identifying whether your blood levels have sufficient nutrients that your body requires. This can be reassuring along your journey, especially if you feel as though you aren't seeing any physical or noticeable results.

Doing blood tests regularly along your journey can benefit you in countless ways, as they can keep you informed on your body. Your blood doesn't lie, as it tells you exactly what it requires from you to make your body holistically healthy and happy. As blood testing is quite popular amongst biohackers, you can find personalized blood testers like InsideTracker, which is catered to biohackers. These are some popular and valuable blood tests you should consider getting done:

- **Complete blood count.** This is a basic and common blood test that records the amount of red blood cells you have, which is crucial, as they transport oxygen and nutrients via your bloodstream. Knowing your red blood cell count can help you understand nutrient deficiencies and delayed healing periods.

- **Cholesterol.** Your cholesterol levels are extremely important to note, as they can be a great indicator of your health. We can often assume that high cholesterol is the only thing to fear, but low cholesterol can be just as dangerous, as it can reduce hormone production, prevent inflammation repair, and create an imbalance of your neurotransmitters. Testing the cholesterol levels in your blood can help you to make healthier decisions for your body.

- **Vitamins and minerals.** You can do specific blood tests to check the levels of vitamins and minerals in your bloodstream. Knowing this information can ensure that you add the right vitamins and minerals to your diet to optimize your health. This can be accomplished through a finger prick test, or a venous blood test, which means you're drawing blood from your veins.

A blood test can be performed at your GP, local doctor's office, or a clinic. These results will tell you everything you need to know, as they provide you with accurate data. It's suggested that you get blood tests done annually to keep up to date with your health stats. If you are truly invested in this information, you could even do blood tests every six months.

Wearable Technology

Using wearable technology like Apple Watches or Fitbits can keep you up to date with your health achievements. A wearable device is something that can monitor and stay with you always, ensuring that biohacking is integrated into your day-to-day life. These are some wearable devices you can explore:

- Apple Watch, Fitbit, or smartwatches
- Glucose monitors
- Sleep monitors

Using wearable technology when exploring new biohacks can also help you determine whether it's working effectively for you. You gather a variety of data such as your heart rate, fitness level, and other health factors.

Cold and Heat Therapy

Who would think using two different extremes of temperature would be an effective form of therapy? Cold therapy is when you use ice baths and cold plunges to improve your muscle recovery and boost your health. You can also explore ice swimming in negative-degree locations to provide you with various health benefits, such as boosted immunity, reduced anxiety and depression, and improved blood circulation.

Heat therapy allows you to explore saunas which can boost your metabolism and immune system. It can be a great solution for pain relief if you're tense from exercise, you've experienced an injury, or even if you're struggling with chronic pain. These two forms of therapy can also provide you with a sense of stress relief.

High Intensity Interval Training (HIIT)

A popular exercise trend for biohacking is HIIT. It has been trending for a while but is currently gaining popularity in the biohacking world. It is all about practicing bursts of intense exercise and then resting. You do different high-intensity exercises within specific intervals.

This form of intense exercise can push your body to its limits, allowing you to withstand intense physical circumstances. HIIT can help you to boost your heart health, burn calories, promote fat loss, and reduce your blood sugar.

Biofeedback

Biofeedback is all about training your body to function optimally. It's a mind-body strategy that allows you to gain more control over your bodily functions, so you can achieve your physical potential. These biofeedback practices study how your body functions, so you can develop practical solutions that improve your health:

- **Brain waves.** This type of biofeedback monitors and studies your brain waves, through the use of an electroencephalograph (EEG), a machine that measures electrical data. An EEG has scalp pads that sense brain waves that showcase different mental states such as stress and anxiety, and your sleep and wake periods.

- **Heart rate.** To study your heart rate, pads are placed on your chest and your wrists. These pads, also connected to an EEG, will measure your heart rate, which can give you a lot of information about your heart health. This data can inform you of your mental state and your fitness level.

- **Breathing.** To receive biofeedback for your breathing capabilities, you will get bands with sensors placed around your chest. The biofeedback equipment will provide you with data that provides you with information on your breathing patterns and breathing rate. This can make you aware of your lung capacity and health, so you know which exercises you need to do to improve your breathing capacity.

To practice biofeedback, you should go to a professional practitioner for the best results. They will use various professional equipment to collect data on your biological information, to determine whether they can create optimal transformations.

Integrating Science Fiction with Reality

What makes biohacking so fascinating is that you're able to explore science fiction in real life. Groundbreaking practices that don't seem like real life can actually improve your quality of life. Discovering how biohackers join the two worlds of science fiction and practicality can inspire you to explore biohacking to its fullest.

Using Artificial Intelligence and Virtual Reality

Bio-sensory hacking is the act of introducing your senses to alternative realities and settings that challenge your mind and cognitive abilities. Artificial intelligence (AI) and virtual reality (VR) are two growing forms of technology that can improve your education, entertainment, therapy, and enrichment.

You can use this technology to explore different realities and life experiences, which can also provide you with a sense of fulfillment and stress relief. VR can be used as a tool for learning, as you can discover facts about life, and informative knowledge, and immerse yourself in the experience of learning. This allows you to enhance your cognitive abilities within the comfort of your own home, as you see the world firsthand and experience visual learning through this advanced innovation!

Artificial intelligence can improve our day-to-day lives, as we are introduced to a more convenient, easier way of living. AI can help with education, learning, and task completion, as you're provided with AI tools that make you more efficient. Having AI bots to talk to for medical, personal, and educational purposes can be extremely educational and beneficial, as you don't have to wait for a human to respond to you.

Aside from AI and VR being enriching for your mental well-being, it can also have a great entertainment factor, as it takes gaming and other forms of entertainment to the next level. Using VR to game or watch certain shows and movies can provide you with a more immersive experience that awakens all of your senses. Remember that spending time doing the things you enjoy can influence you to enjoy life to the fullest!

Cyborg Biohacking

Becoming one with tech can be a scary thought, as it can seem like such an "unknown." We've watched so many movies about technology taking over, but in reality, is cyborg biohacking really a threat to fear? These are some ways cyborg biohacking can make life more effective for us as humans:

- **Cyborg adaptations.** The thought of living forever can potentially become a reality when considering cyborg biohacking. Scientists are looking into replacing human body parts with robotic and technological parts that can enhance the human experience and longevity. Designing new senses is a cyborg biohacking trend that will only expand with time.

- **Bionics.** Some of the best technological and electrical inventions are bionic limbs and body parts, as they complete many individuals who have been in unfortunate accidents or people who were born with physical defects. Bionics ensure that they don't have to live a different or inconvenient life, as they have prosthetic limbs or body parts that allow them to fulfill daily tasks with more ease.

As bionics, technology, and electronics evolve, humans will be able to transform and develop in ways never seen before. Cyborg biotechnology is all about transcending the human body's capabilities, to make life more convenient, increase longevity, and to improve day-to-day functioning.

Nanotechnology

Nanotechnology is about dealing with any technology within 100 nanometers of size, which is extremely small and not visible to the human eye. It's the scientific practice of studying and altering atoms. Nanotechnology is applied in many fields such as food, batteries, and environmental cases, but for biohacking, you'll focus on medical nanotechnology.

Nanotechnology focuses on studying DNA and practicing gene editing within minutes, instead of taking weeks. This technology can help medical professionals treat cancer with more efficiency and a higher success rate. There are numerous nanotechnology experiments that are testing different forms of chemotherapy and how cancerous cells respond to them. Most nanotechnology innovations are in the experimental phase, but as time and technology advances, they will become a reliable practice for biohackers. However, there are some safe nanotechnology approaches you should consider, especially if you have health issues. For example, getting a small device injected into your body that acts as a medical sensor for any issues you may have.

Exploring Human Microchipping

If you want to take connecting with technology to the next level, chipping yourself is something that you can look into. It's a growing trend for biohackers to implant chips in their hands or forearms. The goal is to be intertwined with technology to maximize the potential of understanding and advancing your biological ability.

You may be apprehensive about microchipping, as it can seem like an overwhelming piece of technology, but this isn't a biohack you want to miss out on. These are some benefits of microchipping that prove the advantages it can present you with in your life:

- **Advanced features.** Microchips can process data that no wearable device can interpret, as well as provide convenience. You can make payments with your microchip, meaning you never have to worry about losing your wallet again. It can provide you with access to control your other devices via your chip.

- **Identification.** Human microchipping can also help you to be identified and tracked. Though the sound of being tracked may sound scary, having a microchip can provide you with a lot more safety than you may realize. Your loved ones can locate you, even if all of your devices are stolen or missing. You also never have to worry about losing it! This can be valuable for medical professionals and legal authorities.

- **Medical reasons.** Microchipping can also play a valuable role in the medical system, as it can be used to track critical information on patients in hospitals. This can ensure efficient and ethical practices that will provide life-changing and potentially life-saving results.

These chips and implants can be programmed and fulfill a variety of functions, these are just a few of them. We already make use of wearable devices and cellphones, so why not take it to the next level and experience full benefits from human microchipping?

Evaluating the Potential Benefits and Risks of Advanced Biohacking Techniques

Exploring technological devices and advanced techniques can come with its own pros and cons. It's important to be aware of the risk factors so that you can make the most of advanced biohacking. If you're apprehensive about using technology, knowing how beneficial these biohacking techniques can be for you will motivate you to take advantage of the various resources out there.

Understanding the Potential Benefits

Biohacking isn't always easy, as everyday life gets in the way of your practices and you struggle to stay consistent and accountable. If this is something that is stunting you along your journey, you should consider what advanced biohacking techniques can do for you. The following benefits are what make biohacking gadgets and technology such a great investment:

- **Convenience.** One of the greatest benefits of taking advantage of advanced technology is that you experience a lot of convenience. Life is easier when you have a reliable device at your disposal that you can use wherever and whenever you please. It can make your day-to-day responsibilities a lot more manageable and convenient.

- **Enhancing your progress.** If you're an impatient person who doesn't want to wait to see results in their quality of life, using technology can enhance your progress and help you to achieve your goals and desires at a faster rate. Whether you're using a device to help you sleep, track your daily calories, or motivate you to stay on track with biohacking, you will notice a lot more progress when technology is on your side.

- **Access to more information.** As we discussed previously, it's crucial for you to keep updated with new biohacks and innovations in the market. The best way to accomplish this is by using your devices to stay in the loop. Following well-known biohacking blogs or influencers can keep you up to date while exposing you to some groundbreaking trends that can take your biohacking to the next level.

Technology is continuously evolving, so why not embrace it and take advantage of it, instead of fearing it? You never know how much you can benefit from these positive aspects of technology when you explore everything that is available to you.

Uncovering the Risk Factors

Though biohacking technology is advanced and beneficial, there is also a negative side to it that should be explored. Many people, even biohackers, have concerns about how advanced technology truly is and the negatives it could potentially introduce to our lives. These are some risk factors and cons that you should be aware of when exploring technology devices and gadgets:

- **Being consumed by technology.** Though technological devices can be so effective and valuable for you and your journey, they can also be negative as they consume your time and focus. Instead of spending time on a helpful app to stay organized and accomplish all of your biohacks, you find yourself scrolling through social media and doing things that aren't productive. The next thing you know, four hours have passed and you haven't stopped scrolling through social media apps. It can waste a lot of your time that you could've used to be productive.

- **Depending on your devices.** Though technology is there to make your life easier, you shouldn't find yourself overly dependent on these devices and what they can do for you. This can have the opposite effect of boosting your cognitive abilities, as you find yourself dumbing things down for technology. The first thing you do when you wake up in the morning is look at your phone and the last thing you do before you sleep is spend time on your devices. From this, you'll find your everyday life consumed by technology.

- **Technology taking over our future.** As amazing as technology is for us, the dark side of technology is that it has the ability to completely take over our future. Artificial intelligence, advanced technology, and robotics can take opportunities from workers, as companies are finding more efficient, convenient, and less costly ways of operating. With unemployment rates already increasing, this can cause an unemployment crisis for many countries in the future.

Though these negatives are an unfortunate reality of technology, you shouldn't let this prevent you from pursuing it, as the benefits you can receive are immeasurable. It's all about knowing your limits and having control when using technology. If you know when to stop and give yourself limits, you'll be able to use it wisely and benefit properly without experiencing the risk factors.

Real-World Applications of Biohacking Technologies

Biohacking technologies are used a lot more frequently around us than we may realize. They are designed to make the real world more convenient and efficient. These technologies are shaping our future as individuals and biohackers. Here are some real-world applications of biohacking:

- **Healthcare.** The healthcare system can benefit greatly from biohacking, as it can promote longevity amongst patients and even save lives. Some examples of cutting-edge biohacking technology include biofeedback, as it can prevent and catch medical conditions, and nanotechnology, which can advance medicine.

- **Athletic performance.** Biohacking strategies can be seen through athletes, as they use these techniques to advance their physical capabilities. Athletes can boost their athletic performance through wearable devices that measure their fitness progress, and hot and cold therapy that can speed up their recovery process.

- **Personal wellness.** If you practice habits to ensure your health and well-being, you're most likely applying biohacks to your day-to-day life without even realizing it. If you practice exercises, healthy eating, and technological convenience, you are close to experiencing the next mile with cyborg biohacking and HIIT.

There are various biohacks that surround us in this day and age, as most organizations and communities find ways to integrate technology into their practices. These innovations can be easier to integrate into your life when you realize how practical they are in the real world. These success stories, show you how frequent biohacking truly is:

- **Ross Lynch.** Ross Lynch is a well-known actor, singer, and celebrity who attributes his high-energy performances to biohacking. He swears by techniques like saunas and cold therapy, but his most practiced biohack is intermittent fasting. He practices intermittent fasting while on tour, as it improves his sleep and digestive system, leaving him more energized for his shows.

- **Cristiano Ronaldo.** A famous footballer we all know, Cristiano Ronaldo, also practices biohacks before a big game. When he's leading up to a big game, he introduces sleep intervals to his routine, as he naps up to six times within 24 hours, each nap lasting 90 minutes.

- **Zlatan Ibrahimovic.** Ibrahimovic is an athlete who has taken advantage of what biohacking has to offer. He swears by cold therapy and explores it in the form of cryotherapy, which is a treatment where you're placed in either extremely freezing or hot conditions to eliminate abnormal tissue. This therapy is only performed by professionals. Ronaldo and other famous athletes are also known to use it for muscle recovery.

Let these stories inspire you to make biohacking a part of your story to success. Whatever your goals may be in life, using biohacking as a tool will help you to get there faster!

Chapter 9:

Implementing Biohacking in Your Daily Life

Biohacking isn't a temporary fix, as it's a lifestyle that can completely transform your way of living. It's time for you to implement these hacks into your day-to-day lifestyle so that you can make the most of biohacking. Make the changes in your life that you need, so you can live the lifestyle you so deeply desire. The more you implement biohacking in your daily life, the easier these strategies and techniques will become for you!

Practical Tips for Integrating Biohacking into Your Daily Routine

It can be challenging to completely transform your way of life when you're so used to a specific daily routine. You don't know how to seamlessly integrate this change into your daily routine so that it's something you continuously stick to each day. You're more likely to stick to a certain routine or habits when they become a part of everyday life for you.

Build Your Biohacking Lifestyle

Now that you've discovered all of the valuable hacks and methods you can use to unlock your biological potential, it's time for you to build a biohacking lifestyle that you're happy with. You're not just integrating these habits into your day-to-day life, as you are dedicating yourself to a completely transformed lifestyle. This can be really overwhelming, so to have more guidance and control, follow these steps to build your biohacking lifestyle:

- **Fix your sleeping schedule.** Start off by adjusting your sleep schedule. You can't focus on this journey, make necessary changes, and positively adapt your habits and lifestyle if you're drained from insufficient sleep. Calculate what time you have to be up every morning, and from this information, you can determine what time you should be sleeping every night.

- **Transform your diet.** It's time to go to your kitchen and change your diet. What you have in your cupboards and fridge will ultimately determine what your day-to-day diet looks like. You need to get rid of all of the unhealthy and toxic food that is setting you back and make a list of all the healthy replacements you can purchase when you go grocery shopping. Try out one of the diets from Chapter 2 that you're most excited about and identify how much each diet can help you to achieve the best results. Cut out the toxic foods or habits that have been setting your diet back.

- **Investigate supplements and advancements.** It's now time to investigate so you can find any supplements or advancements that can make your experience with biohacking more successful. Go through the chapter on supplements and identify what type of supplements you need to solve particular issues in your life. Consider other advancements like technology and devices that can make your journey easier and more effective.

- **Participate in self-care.** To succeed in biohacking, you need to look after your physical and mental well-being. You need to look after your well-being to ensure that you become the best version of yourself. Take the necessary breaks your body requires, look after yourself, and engage in self-care activities that nourish and nurture your mind, body, and soul. When you look after your holistic being, you'll be able to excel more on your journey.

- **Introduce exercise to your lifestyle.** One of the main components of a successful biohacking lifestyle is exercising regularly. Finding an exercise that you enjoy the most while being able to push yourself physically will allow you to achieve both physical and mental growth. Setting fitness goals and working toward them each day will be the best thing you can do for your health in the long run!

- **Habit formation.** Once you've started to adapt to biohacks, it's important for you to work on transforming these hacks into habits. You'll only truly benefit from biohacking when you turn these healthy habits into your daily routine. It takes a while for a task, behavior, or practice to become a habit, so it's crucial that you give yourself the time you need to create this routine for yourself. Continuous practice and effort will allow you to create these biohacking habits that lead you to success.

Once you've conquered each one of these steps, you'll be on your way to achieving a biohacking lifestyle that allows you to thrive from the inside out. It can seem overwhelming at first, as there are so many hacks to be mindful of to ensure a successful biohacking lifestyle, but the most effective way for you to approach this is by tackling each aspect of your life one at a time. As you go through these guided steps, tick each task off so that you can be aware of the amazing progress you're making.

Overcoming Common Challenges and Obstacles

Unfortunately, this journey won't be completely perfect and flawless, as you will find yourself experiencing common challenges and obstacles along the way. It's important for you to be mentally prepared for this so that you don't feel negative feelings toward yourself that make you want to give up.

Give it Time

When you're starting with biohacking, you may find that you don't receive the immediate results you may have expected. It takes time for biohacking to have a significant impact on our life, as you need to fully commit your time and effort to performing the most suitable hacks for you. Give yourself the necessary time to see results. This will ensure that you stay dedicated to the journey regardless of the obstacles you may face.

We can often all be impatient to see results but be kind and patient with yourself. Believe in yourself and your abilities to transform your biological capabilities. You and your body are capable of far more than you even realize, so give it time and watch the magic happen!

Trying New Biohacks

If you've given your biohacking routine some time and you still aren't seeing the results you desire, you may want to consider trying out some new biohacks. It's important for you to switch up your biohacking routine to suit you, as not all biohacks work for everyone.

It can feel disheartening when you start this journey, and you aren't receiving the results you want or feeling comfortable with the changes you're making. Instead of being disappointed and giving up on biohacking, it's important for you to try new biohacks. Keep trying new healthy and enriching habits until you discover what works for you. This may require a long journey of trial and error, but it will be entirely worth it in the end.

Adjusting to Change

Change is never easy, especially when you're letting go of habits that make you really happy. Biohacking can introduce you to a lot of change at once, which can be a massive hurdle to cross. Once you learn how to tackle change, you'll be able to make the necessary transformations that provide you with a long and healthy life:

- **Pace yourself.** If you know that you're not good with change, it may be a valuable idea to pace yourself with this process. Instead of changing every habit and routine at once, start introducing yourself to change slowly and gradually. You can start off by introducing exercise to your lifestyle, proceed to cut out toxic habits like smoking, and you can then transform your diet. Slowly but surely tackling every biohack will introduce you to change in a much more manageable manner.

- **Replace your comfortable coping mechanisms.** When we come from an unhealthy lifestyle that isn't advancing our health or well-being, we can find ourselves depending on toxic coping mechanisms. For example, you may use unhealthy foods as a coping mechanism, as they provide you with a sense of comfort and help you to forget about your worries in life. When you take that coping mechanism away, it can make it challenging for you to get through day-to-day life. This is why you should find healthy replacements for these habits that help your change feel a little less foreign. If you rely on unhealthy foods, find some healthy snacks you enjoy replacing them with. If you smoke to relieve stress, try deep breathing exercises to manage your stress.

- **Be patient.** Once again, we're going to emphasize the need for you to be patient with yourself. It's imperative for you to give yourself time to adjust to change because it may seem strange at first to have a different routine, but as each day goes on, it becomes more normal and familiar. Change becomes a way of life once you're patient with yourself and this journey. Don't give up before change begins to feel like a normal way of life for you.

When you successfully adjust to the change of biohacking, you will feel more comfortable and committed to this journey. Everything you do feels right, as it just feels like regular daily life for you. Though this biohacking journey may feel overwhelming now, once you become comfortable, your future self will be thanking you greatly for your consistency and patience.

Resisting Tempting Bad Habits

Something that could be setting you back in your biohacking journey is being tempted by unhealthy habits, foods, and a way of life that isn't good for you and your progress. You crave bad foods, and unhealthy habits, and you wish to be lazy, instead of being proactive with biohacks. It can be especially challenging to resist temptation when you're surrounded by people who aren't living a healthy lifestyle. Here are some effective ways you can resist temptation along this journey:

- **Reward yourself.** Rewarding yourself frequently can prevent you from indulging in things that aren't good for you. When you allow yourself to have a treat every now and then, you'll be less tempted by negative habits or foods, as you aren't restricting yourself entirely. Positive reinforcement can also keep you encouraged to do more and stay consistent, as it makes you realize how much of an accomplishment staying consistent is. Every time you spend two weeks being consistent with your biohacks, you can reward yourself with one of your favorite treats.

- **Staying focused.** The best way to resist temptation is by staying focused along this journey. The big question for you may be, "How does one stay focused?". It can seem impossible to stay focused, but you need to be able to master this so that you can showcase consistency along your journey. A great way for you to remain focused each day is by keeping your bigger picture in mind. Realizing that you're practicing biohacking to achieve your dream goals and long healthy lifestyle, makes all of the strenuous hard work and consistency worth it. Whenever you find yourself being distracted by tempting bad habits, remind yourself of the bigger picture that has brought you here.

- **Keep yourself accountable.** If you want to turn these biohacking practices into everyday habits, you need to be able to keep yourself accountable and take responsibility for your actions. Set goals and biohacking tasks for yourself each day and ensure that you reach them no matter what is happening in your life. Whenever you indulge in a negative habit, be aware of it and prevent yourself from repeating the same mistake. As you continuously hold yourself accountable for what you do on your agenda and what you neglect, you're more likely to stick to a healthy routine. You may find it valuable to tell your friends and family about this journey, as they can also help you to stay accountable.

- **Forgiving yourself for mistakes.** If you do happen to make mistakes and binge eat that cake you weren't supposed to or get a few hours of sleep because you were up all night gaming, it's important not to be too hard on yourself. It's okay to make mistakes and be a little inconsistent with your biohacking routine, in fact, it's normal for this to happen. What's important is that you don't get caught up in guilt and continue the negative behavior of giving up. When you do something that goes against your new biohacking routine, accept it, realize you were wrong, and forgive yourself. This will allow you to move on and make better decisions.

Unfortunately, temptation will always surround you when you're trying to transform and introduce health and prosperity into your life. All that matters is how you handle it. It will be a lot more manageable for you to stay consistent when you feel more in control and as though you're able to avoid the tempting negative habits that could hold your progress back.

Strengthening Your Mind and Body Connection

If you feel as though you're really struggling with your biohacking journey, as you aren't receiving all of the results you desired and you find it impossible to stay focused and in control, it's time for you to strengthen your mind and body connection. When it comes to biohacking, it's all about advancing your biological strength and abilities, while healing and restoring your mental and cognitive capabilities. These are some ways you can work on strengthening your mind and body:

- **Yoga.** Practicing activities like yoga can help to strengthen that mind-body connection. You can explore various intensities of yoga to experience different results, as it can also be a great form of exercise. When you practice various yoga positions, you challenge your body to achieve greater strength, stability, and inner peace. Your mind and body work as one, as you perform intricate positions that showcase your strength and resilience. It can take a lot of practice and willpower to get where you want with yoga, which helps you to work from within yourself to find the inner strength to accomplish your yoga goals.

- **Engaging with your five senses.** A great way for you to achieve a deeper mind and body connection is by engaging all five of your senses and utilizing them accordingly. Take some time from your day to practice this engaging exercise with items around you wherever you are. Close your eyes and draw your attention and awareness to the sounds happening around you. Do you hear cars, people talking, or birds chirping? Smell the aromas that surround you and specifically identify each one. You can then open your eyes and take a look at everything around you. What objects are around you that you've never noticed before? Pick one unique object to touch and observe through its texture and purpose. If you have anything edible around you, you can also explore your sense of taste, by giving it a try and identifying all the different flavors within this food item. This simple mindfulness activity can allow you to bring your attention to the present moment, as it brings all of your senses alive, as you engage your mind simultaneously.

If you truly commit yourself to a biohacking routine, you will find that your mind and body connection really strengthens, as you are practicing healthy habits that nourish this connection. Your healthy eating allows your body to thrive and your mind to become sharper than ever. As you explore rest and recovery, you're able to strengthen that nurturing bond with your mind and body. When you relax and practice stress management, you're able to focus on that special connection between your mind and body.

Conclusion

Biohacking is the harmony of using all of these strategies and techniques together. It can seem overwhelming at first, as there are so many habits you must adjust and change in your life, but once you learn how to successfully tackle each aspect of your life, you will thrive in health, longevity, and prosperity.

Fearing the future, how you may age, and the realities of health struggles and stressors can be daunting. You want to thrive in your youth forever, but even in your present state, you experience health issues and a level of unfitness that makes you unsatisfied with yourself and your life. Your cognitive functioning is not where it needs to be for you to accomplish all of your wildest dreams. These are all common problems people experience before they fully embrace biohacking. Once you practice biohacking, you will discover how you're able to tackle and transform all of these issues.

Biohacking is about completely transforming your lifestyle, by integrating some effective biohacks within your day-to-day life. The way you view food transforms, as you don't think about it as a means to end your hunger, but rather as something that will nourish and enrich your mind and body. This makes you more mindful of the foods you put into your body. You ensure that you get all of your macro and micronutrients onto each plate, and you enrich your body with supplements and high-quality foods that leave your gut happy and healthy.

You'll also integrate healthy habits into your daily lifestyle like exercising regularly, learning how to manage your stress, and most importantly, enhancing your cognitive abilities. Being able to manage your stress will not only help you to live a long and healthy life, but it will also drastically improve your quality of life, as you don't let your worries consume you on a daily basis. Regular exercise can help you to manage your stress, as well as help you to reach the physical goals that you've been longing for. Enhancing your cognitive capabilities will allow you to advance in your career, and personal life, and you'll build confidence in yourself and your mental capabilities.

Technology is the future, so find ways to integrate technology into your day-to-day life so that your biohacking journey becomes easier. Use your devices to benefit you, instead of using them as distractions that cause you to be less productive. Do your research and find some of the most fascinating technological innovations that can make your biohacking life easier and more convenient. When buying technological devices, don't forget to shop and invest in items wisely, as you want to spend your money on devices that will last you a lifetime of happiness.

It's also important for you to remember that it will take time for you to notice results from biohacking, as it's not something that is instant. Be patient with yourself and find resilience when you meet hurdles along the way of your journey. There will be learning curves, as well as there will be moments where you just don't feel like practicing biohacks. What's important is that you persevere through these feelings and embrace biohacking in its entirety.

With time and practice, you will discover how biohacking can transform your life. It's time to think for your future self and see how much it benefits the longevity and health of your life. Aging no longer has to be something you fear or dread, as you get to enjoy this stage of your life. You move around independently and live a long and healthy life that fills you with satisfaction. Great health provides you with a sense of freedom that you can't pay for.

Remember that this is your journey, so you need to treat it like that. You can follow popular biohackers or practice other peoples' biohacking routines meticulously, but you're probably not going to achieve the results you want. You need to personalize this routine for your own mind and body. Experiment with yourself, practice trial and error, and discover what works specifically for you. The more you play around with biohacks, the more likely you are to find a routine that is suitable for you. Trust the process. Don't be afraid to adapt biohacks to your body, while still keeping them effective.

It's time for you to look out for your future self, by practicing all of the biohacking it takes for you to achieve the lifestyle and health that you desire for yourself. Start making those small changes in your life and discover how much it can benefit you holistically. Before you know it, you'll be a skilled biohacker with remarkable health and satisfaction with your lifestyle. It's up to you to make this lifetime the best and longest one it can be! What biohacks are you going to try first?

Continue Your Journey with the Biohacking Planner

Congratulations on reaching the end of this transformative journey. Your dedication to holistic well-being has brought you here, and now the path to biohacking mastery extends even further.

As you embark on your personalized journey, we want to express our deepest appreciation for choosing to explore the empowering insights within these pages. We hope you've discovered valuable tips and insights that ignite your path to peak performance and well-being.

To further enhance your experience, we invite you to download our exclusive Biohacking planner via the QR code. This essential tool is your companion in optimizing every facet of your life, empowering you to sculpt a future of unwavering and relentless fulfilment.

Your feedback is invaluable. If you've enjoyed this book, we encourage you to leave a review to help others seeking similar transformative experiences. Your support can inspire and guide fellow seekers on their path to empowerment.

Thank you for choosing to prioritize your well-being. Your journey toward unlimited energy, unyielding focus, and unshakable vitality begins now.

Good luck in your holistic health journey!

Olivia Rivers

References

Bedosky, L. (2022, May 31). *What are essential oils? A complete guide on aromatherapy and its potential health benefits.* Everyday Health. https://www.everydayhealth.com/wellness/what-are-essential-oils-a-complete-guide-on-aromatherapy-and-its-potential-health-benefits/

Bertone, H. J., & Hoshaw.C. (2021, November 5). *Which type of meditation is right for me?* Healthline; Healthline Media. https://www.healthline.com/health/mental-health/types-of-meditation#mindfulness-meditation

Bhanote, M. (2022, October 17). *What to know about biohacking.* MedicalNewsToday. https://www.medicalnewstoday.com/articles/biohacking

Biofeedback. (n.d.). Cleveland Clinic. https://my.clevelandclinic.org/health/treatments/13354-biofeedback

8 biohacking trends to look out for in 2023. (n.d.). TheLifeCo. https://www.thelifeco.com/en/blog/8-biohacking-trends-to-look-out-for-in-2023

Gotter, A. (2023, March 22). *8 breathing exercises to try when you feel anxious.* Healthline. https://www.healthline.com/health/breathing-exercises-for-anxiety

Gunnars, K. (2023, August 29). *Intermittent fasting 101 — the ultimate beginner's guide.* Healthline.

https://www.healthline.com/nutrition/intermittent-fasting-guide#methods

Jennings, K.-A. (2023, January 23). *11 best foods to boost your brain and memory.* Healthline. https://www.healthline.com/nutrition/11-brain-foods

Knudsen, M. (2022, November 18). *What Is Biohacking? How to get started and the science behind it.* InsideTracker. https://blog.insidetracker.com/what-is-biohacking

Kraft, A., & Carstensen, M. (2023, March 17). *7 popular supplements that may have hidden dangers.* Everyday Health. https://www.everydayhealth.com/news/supplements-risks-every-women-should-know/

McPherson, G. (2022, November 5). *4 supplements you should actually be taking, according to a dietitian.* EatingWell. https://www.eatingwell.com/article/8009984/supplements-you-should-consider-taking/

Nye, C. (2018, December 5). *Biohacker: Meet the people "hacking" their bodies.* BBC News. https://www.bbc.com/news/technology-46442519

Penner, E. (n.d.). *What supplements should you not take together?* ELO Smart Nutrition. https://www.elo.health/answers/what-supplements-should-you-not-take-together/

Richmond, C. (n.d.). *Supplements: What you really need.* WebMD. https://www.webmd.com/vitamins-and-supplements/ss/slideshow-supplements-myths-facts

Saturn by GHC. (2022, July 5). *3 biohacking myths, debunked in 3 minutes.* Saturn by GHC. https://saturn.health/blogs/news/3-biohacking-myths-debunked-in-3-minutes

Stibich, M. (2022, September 24). *10 best brain games to keep your mind sharp.* Verywell Mind. https://www.verywellmind.com/top-websites-and-games-for-brain-exercise-2224140

Streit, L. (2023, July 13). *Micronutrients: Types, functions, benefits and more.* Healthline. https://www.healthline.com/nutrition/micronutrients #types-and-functions

Velazquez, R. (2023, July 7). *Nootropics for beginners – quick start guide to 100% brainpower.* Mind Lab Pro®. https://www.mindlabpro.com/blogs/nootropics/nootropics-beginners

Printed in Great Britain
by Amazon